WALK AWAY ACHES & PAINS

3 HOURS OF CEU'S FOR HEALTH PARTITIONERS

A Self-Empowerment Guide to be Pain-Free from Shins Splints, Low Back Pain, Plantar Fasciitis, Achilles Tendonitis, Falling Arches, Knee Pain, Scoliosis, Sciatica, and many other leg and back issues.

——— Written and Illustrated by ———
JACOB CALDWELL, LMT

©Copyright 2011-2019 by Exoflow, LLC 5429 Russell Ave NW #300, Seattle WA 98107. All rights reserved. No part of this publication may be reproduced by any means or for any reason without the consent of the publisher. The information contained herein is obtained from sources believed to be reliable, but its accuracy cannot be guaranteed.

All material in this publication is provided for information only and may not be construed as medical advice or instruction. No action or inaction should be taken based solely on the contents of this publication: instead, readers should consult appropriate health professionals on any matter relating to their health and well-being. The information and opinions provided in this publication are believed to be accurate and sound, based on the best judgement available to the author, but readers who fail to consult with appropriate health authorities assume the risk of any injuries. The publisher is not responsible for errors or omissions. The material in this report has not been approved by the American Medical Association (AMA) or the FDA. The products and materials discussed are not intended to diagnose, treat, cure, or prevent any disease.

Walk Away Aches & Pains

A Self-Empowerment Guide to be Pain-Free from

Low Back Pain
Shin Splints
Sciatica
Achilles Tendonitis

Plantar Fasciitis
Falling Arches
Knee Pain
Scoliosis
and any other leg issues

Written & Illustrated

By

Jacob Caldwell, LMT, CPT

Copyright 2011-2019

Introduction xi

Chapter One 1

Range of Motion (ROM) of the Ankles is equal to Range of Motion of the HIP

Chapter Two 11

Toes Forward

Chapter Three 25

The 4 Step Points

Chapter Four 37

Grip the Ground – No more Falling Arches

Chapter Five 43

The 3 Axes

Chapter Six   51

Walking Activates Health

Chapter Seven   67

Walking Incorrectly Effects Posture

Chapter Eight   79

The Core

Chapter Nine   83

Posture – Putting it all together

Chapter Ten   89

Not all Pain is created equal

The Case for how Osteoarthritis is Created

Chapter Eleven   117

Mental Manifesting

Chapter Twelve 123

Shoes – The Good, Bad, and the Funny Looking

Chapter Thirteen 137

Sports and Recreation

Chapter Fourteen 141

Solutions & Exercises for Superior Walking Health

Chapter Fifteen 151

What is Water?

Chapter Sixteen 167

The StretchFlex Technique

A Stretch a day keeps the Surgeon away

Notes	175
Index	185
Other Books by Jacob	191
Continuing Education Credits	197
Walking Demo Videos	198

The awareness of this material has giving me more awareness of how I place my foot in my yoga practice. I am now flexing more of my inner legs which is making my back stronger and a lot of my back pain has gone away.

-Sandra Lantz

This information has blown me away. I had given up running due to my plantar fasciitis and thought I will never run again. The information and exercises in the "Falling Arches" Chapter gave me the inspiration that I would be able to run again. After 5 months I am running like I used to.

-John Hanson

I have been receiving massage from Jacob for over a year now. I came in having chronic achilles pain, a sore knee, and a low back pain on my right side. I was taking ibuprofen every other day for the pain. Jacob offered advice from this book towards my issues. He advised that may Achilles issues is due to not lifting my foot enough. I tried this and after a few months and I have not had the pain again for a while. I worked the walking technique some more and my low back pain and knee pain gradually resided. I also tried the advice of gripping the ground to resolve my falling arches. After a few months there is a visual difference in that the integrity of my arches have gone back to their original position. I told my boyfriend about the advice of how to take care of his low back pain. We massaged his calves and did the walking technique and his low back pain has greatly lessened. I have not totally mastered the walking technique and sometimes I forget, but when I do feel one of the old pains, I just use it as a reminder to "Walk Correctly" again and the pain goes away. I haven't taken ibuprofen for months. I feel stronger in my legs and I am happy to learn how to resolve my own body pains.

-Christina Coleman

Introduction

Empower your health with knowledge and resolve your own ailments.

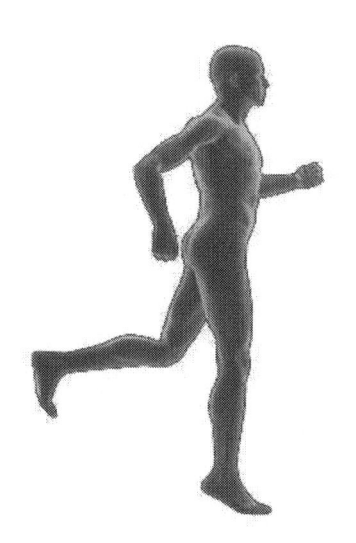

WARNING: This how to walk technique is for people who want to empower their own self-healing and take control of their life. Do not read any further if you have a closed mind and are looking for excuses as to why you are not getting better. Without an open mind, upcoming text may be very disturbing and frightening to you. If one reads and carries out these techniques you may become healthier, happier, and not have any more excuses to use. This information is for perseverant and personally responsible people only. You have been Warned! Good Luck!

How to "Walk Away Aches & Pains", is so simple of a statement it doesn't make sense. "Of course, I know how to walk; I've been doing it since I was born." Yes, you have been. What we have also could have been doing is creating chronic inflammatory ailments at the same time by not walking correctly. In sports, technique will win out over strength most of the time.

As a Massage Therapist, my focus and passion has always been to empower people to heal themselves. Healer means "To Inspire", Doctor means "To Teach", and in my book if you are not being taught or inspired by your practitioner on how to resolve your issue, then this is called failure. Failure in medicine and therapy is when you repeat the same practice and achieve very little progress with the same level of pain for the client. The same definition applies to "Insanity" – doing the same thing repeatedly and expecting a different result.

I have always been curious on how an injury occurs. It always seems like a game to me in finding the mystery to how the pain got there. Often many people do not know what the source of their pain is and usually practitioners don't bother to find out. It is imperative to find out how that hip pain got there. Was it from a fall 10 years ago or is it from walking your dog every day? If we can prevent an incorrect activity that is causing us pain, then we can administer the correct healing procedure. However, we need the person to stop hurting themselves so that they can progressively heal. If the person is currently hurting themselves daily it is quite difficult to have an effective treatment plan.

The most profound and preventable injury that I see is that people do not walk correctly due to an usual walk or foot position[1]. As a society, we don't really walk anymore. We walk to the bathroom, to the car, down the hall, but now we rarely walk a mile or 2 to work or to the store. Sometimes I will hear, "I had to park 3 blocks away to get here!" If you have trouble walking 3 blocks, you need to walk those 3 blocks.

We are such a technological society that we have stomped on Nature for egotistical technology. We think an MRI and surgery is going to help us with our knee issue when really it comes down to flexing a muscle correctly. We think technology is going to save us from everything, but if we can listen to Nature it has all the solutions already. The problem is we must listen to Nature and accept things are easy, which is the hard part.

I have seen many different pain issues such as arthritis, scoliosis, plantar fasciitis, bursitis, inflamed joints, ACL/MCL tears, shin splints, falling arches, tight IT bands, bunions, low back pain, chronic neck pain, and one leg shorter than the other. As far as I am concerned these issues all must do with one thing: HOW YOUR FOOT CONTACTS THE GROUND. If you have ever constructed a house you would know that the leveling of the foundation is an important part of the building process, otherwise you will have crooked windows, walls, and roofs. So, goes the same with the body.

The full range of motion of the leg and foot must be exercised; otherwise, if one continually skips parts of the steps it will be like a house on a slowly sinking foundation. Soon you will have chronic issues above the waist and no matter what kind of therapy you do, the issue never resolves and continually reappears. Usually where the pain is, is not the problem, but the symptom. If the window is crooked it has nothing to do with the window itself; it is the crooked foundation and the same thing happens with the body. Often crooked hips and low back pain must do with the simple technique of not flexing your big toe. You can rub that back all you want but if you do not flex that toe, your back is going to keep hurting for a long time.

There have been many devices like orthotics, ointments, and surgeries but all of these are temporary solutions. If you do not flex that foot correctly nothing will change. I have had people lay on my massage bed and they think all they need is for me to rub that spot and it will be gone. And then I have to apologize and say, "This session is only effective for inspiring you on how to heal" and "you sir/ma'am need to flex your foot properly."

Unfortunately, Walking naturally is not an easy thing to master at first and takes a lot of discipline. Breaking habits is very difficult but the rewards to being able to heal yourself and prevent further injury are quite empowering. I like to think, if I was thrown out into the forest, would I have to need anything? I don't want to have to depend on needing something like pharmaceuticals, orthotics, or syringes. I want to be truly health empowered with self-knowledge. After learning to be more conscious of how you walk, you are going to have to ask yourself, "If I can heal this what else can I do?" Answer: Everything!

At first, learning how to walk again requires a lot of thinking about your feet and can seem overwhelming and that is why I have broken the steps up so that you can focus on one thing at a time. It is tough to do them all at once but if you can do one, you can do the next.

There are many ways to create low back pain or any issue of the body. There is no absolute issue that will guarantee to create an issue or disorder. Often issues are created to a variety of missteps. So, it is up to you, the person with the pain to observe yourself and use this book as a guide or inspiration to apply any of these suggestions to you. This book is meant as a general guide to help inspire you to see that you can resolve your issues yourself.

Chapter One

Range of Motion (ROM) of the Ankles is equal to Range of Motion of the Hip

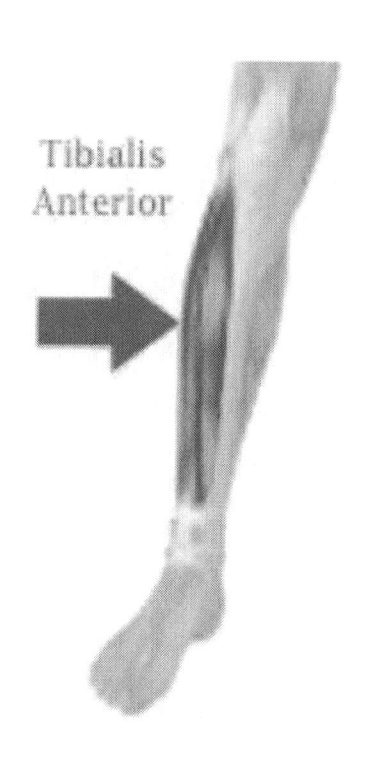

Tibialis Anterior

Flexibility and exercising the full ROM ("range of motion") of any appendage should be a major goal to focus on.[1] This is what I like about yoga; it puts you in positions you would not ordinarily get into yourself. While yoga helps to tone and strengthen joints while utilizing full range of motion[2]; the key to mastering this walking technique is to practice body awareness and foot presence.

I have observed that most people's ankles are stiff and are stuck at the 90-degree ankle. When the leg takes a step forward, the front of the foot should be lifted upwards as well, while making sure to hit the heel on the ground first and not be flat-footed. You should feel your tibialis anterior working very hard and if it "hurts" you are doing it right. [3]

Two kinds of Pain

In reference to working your muscle till it "hurts". There are two kinds of pain. Hurting yourself that causes inflammation and fatiguing a muscle that is not in shape. I am referring to working on a muscle till if fatigues. When one has not worked a muscle correctly and then starts exercising it in a new way, just like any new exercise it takes a little while to get that muscle in shape. What to watch out for is hurting yourself. Injury and muscle fatigue can almost feel the same. The difference is that injuring yourself will result in inflammation and constant ongoing pain for days.[4] Muscle fatigue will hurt more in the moment and should not have a lingering pain response later.[5] Eventually when you work this muscle into shape the pain will gradually go away because your muscle has become stronger. If it does not go away, then you may be injuring yourself or aggravating an old injury that has not repaired yet.

Too Tight, Too Hard, & Overstretched

Often in this book I will be referring to muscles being too tight or too hard. This will be regarding a muscle that is doing too much work and not enough rest. When a muscle is worked too hard and not receiving enough healing therapy or stretching, it will become hard and tight. If it is worked constantly in one direction it may stay in that position and harden.

Every joint has an appendage and a muscle group that will pull the appendage in one direction and an opposing muscle group will pull the appendage in the opposite direction. This can be seen as a tug-o-war if they are not of equal strength. If one muscle group is pulling one way all the time, then the other group will be pulled along with it. The group doing most of the work will become shortened and stay in this position and It will gradually become tight and hard. The opposite muscle group will become elongated and will be pulled towards the shortened muscle group. This opposite muscle group will begin to be overstretched and out of position. Because it is now being compromised by being pulled in a direction that is unnatural it will begin to tighten as well. An overstretched muscle group will often be the group that exudes the most pain because it is being pulled off the bone at the tendon. Muscles have some give but tendons do not. This is why most of the pin-point inflamed pain areas are located where the tendon connects to the bone. The overstretched muscle group will harden in order to protect itself. So, the root cause of such pains is initially from the overworked muscles group that shortens into itself. However, it exudes very little pain, unless it is pressed on, like what would happen in a massage therapy session. With every out of balanced opposing muscle group, to really resolve the issue both opposing muscle groups need to receive therapy. Just working on the painful area is not enough and may never resolve. We must lengthen the shortened overworked muscle group and shorten and flex the overstretched muscle group. This will be a repeating theme in this book which may resolve many of your chronic leg, foot, and back issues.

Most posture related pain areas and chronic sports injuries are really about foot placement technique. Pain is often created because we are not paying attention to ourselves. This book will provide you with a detail look on how we flex our bodies and that the main cause of many musculoskeletal issues is due to repeatedly compromising body technique. So, to the key to resolving pain, is if we can pay a little more attention to how we move our bodies we can resolve almost anything ourselves.

Increasing the Range of Motion of the Ankle

A major part people miss is the moment before your heel hits the ground. Engaging your tibialis anterior muscle is the muscle that lifts your foot. This action opens your foot to later "catch" the ground (more about this in the "Gripping the Ground" Chapter).

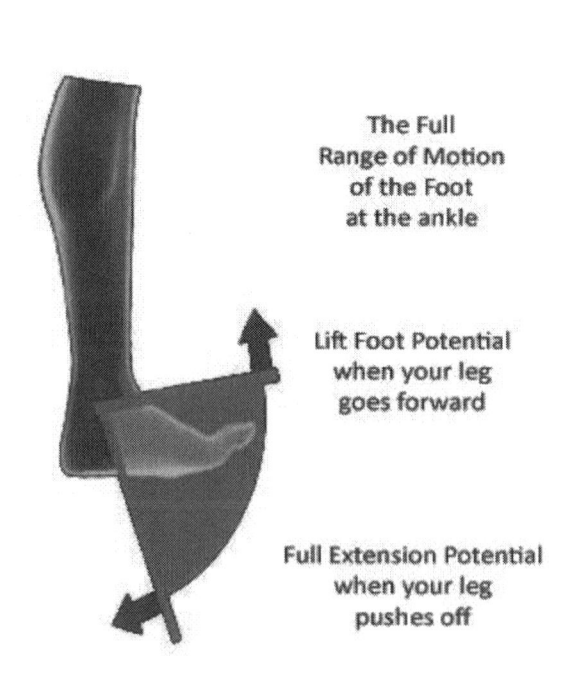

The Full
Range of Motion
of the Foot
at the ankle

Lift Foot Potential
when your leg
goes forward

Full Extension Potential
when your leg
pushes off

When you lift the foot an inch or so more upwards, this will allow your leg to move farther forward in its stride. People with hip issues and tight IT Bands often fall into this category. (IT Band is located on the outside of the leg between the knee and hip.) If one is NOT lifting their foot and allowing their leg to move forward, you will be causing the front of your hip to become atrophied and tight. The joint will become hard and then water and blood will have a difficult time circulating through that muscle. This will make your joint less maneuverable and may make it susceptible to being injured later. Tight muscles are like glass and if jarred suddenly they "shatter". Having your muscles and joints lucid and flexible with a full range of motion will help keep them more tolerable to outer circumstances.

It is good to massage your tibialis anterior to help loosen up the ankle. Hold the muscle and flex your foot up and down. Flex into the muscle while pressing into it. Continue to press into it while stretching it

Holding the Tibialis Anterior

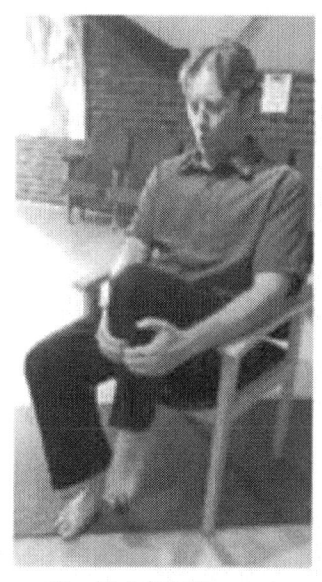

Pushing Down 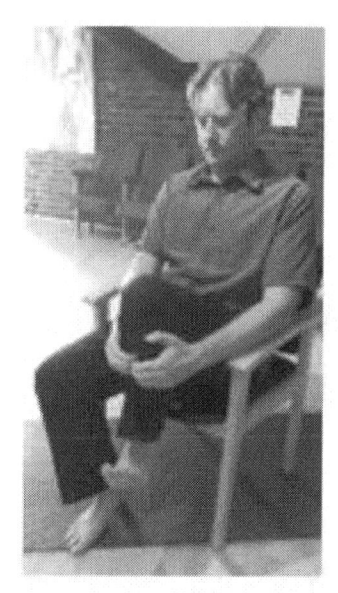   Lifting Up

downwards. This is a bit of the StretchFlex Technique, to be learned at the end of this book.

A condition that can be caused by not lifting the Tibialis Anterior enough is achilles **tendonitis** or tendonosis.[6] People who have this issue may be leaning backwards and the weight of their body is held up by the back of their legs. So, the calves and hamstrings will become overworked and very tight. People with tight hamstrings may be standing this way.

Symptoms of achilles tendon injuries usually include:

- Pain along the back of your foot, pain above your heel or pain at the sides of the ankle bone.
- Throbbing when moving the heel or ankle, especially when lifting the heel and standing on the toes. Some experience severe pain the day after exercising.
- Developing stiffness, swelling, inflamed tissue, thickening and tenderness near the heel.
- Limited range of motion in the ankle or heel.
- Sometimes hearing unusual noises when moving the tendon, such as snapping or popping sounds.[7]

In my research achilles tendonitis is caused by not stretching, too much repetition, overtraining, or having conditions that cause joint deterioration and inflammation.[8] These are all causes that can affect any appendage. To create a part of your body that is stiff like the achilles, one must be doing the same motion for a long period of time. With constant repetition over time there is going to be a breakdown especially if restful therapies or stretching is not used to balance the body.[9]

Usually people will injure themselves when they are involved in a different or new activity. I have seen many times in my practice a professional computer user injures their back because they are moving boxes from one office to another. They normally do not lift boxes, but they push a mouse button all day. There mouse pushing arm is what they use often and so those muscles are tight. But when those same muscles must be flexed in a different direction they are easier to tear. When a muscle becomes tight and not warmed up it can easily be injured. Often what people experience is a "pulled muscle". If you are walking like a robot, which is walking very stiff because you pulled that muscle. Depending on severity, you may be doing the "robot" for a week or 2. You have pulled the muscle, tendon, or a nerve and have now caused a lot of inflammation.[10] The achilles or any foot muscle is carrying a lot of weight and can be asked to perform a lot of activities from different angles. It is important for your feet to be flexible and pliable.

"The concept of long-lasting static posture runs contrary to how the body functions. Sped up video studies have shown that our bodies are always indulging in subtle or gross movements to ensure that one precise posture is NOT held for prolonged periods, thereby ensuring that stresses are not imposed upon the same physical structures in the same way. Even in sporting and other complex movement situations, the same external movement pattern may be produced by different musculoskeletal and neuromuscular strategies, so that the idea of an invariant, highly stable single posture is misleading."

-Mel Siff, Ph.D.

Each muscle has a function and in a walking stride there will be a different muscle used for each part of the foot hitting the ground. The body is designed for one muscle to engage an action while the opposite muscle is relaxing and being stretched. At the beginning of the walking stride the tibialis anterior is lifting the foot up and at the end of the stride the gastrocnemius (calve) is levering the foot down. Nature has already established balance and equilibrium for us. Problems arise when we go out of this balance.

So, if one has achilles tendonitis it could be due to using the gastrocnemius too much and not enough of its counterpart the tibialis anterior being flexed the other direction. When a muscle becomes tight it is because it has been used too much in one direction for a long period time and rarely goes in the other direction.[11] This imbalance may lead to people's posture becoming off-center. This can lead to slumping with the shoulders rolling forward or the hip protruding forward.

Increasing the Range of Motion of the Hip

This part of the walking naturally technique is important because the flexibility of the ankle will dictate the pliability of the rest of the body. If your ankle is stiff it is likely the rest of your body will be stiff. The flexibility of the hip depends on the flexibility of the ankle. If the Tibialis Anterior is stiff due to not being used, the front of the hip will also be stiff. When you lift the foot up you will take a longer stride which will engage the front of your hip. The front hip muscles oversee flexing your leg forward. You can't have a loose hip and tight ankles. Only lucid ankles can make a loose hip. So, if you do not lift that foot you will not be able to flex the front of your hip. Hip issues, either front, back, or side, will be linked to the angle that the foot engages the ground and the muscles flexed in the foot and leg. Therefore, the range of motion of the ankle will be directly tied to the range of motion of the hip. If you have a hip issue start to look at how your foot hits the ground. Often with the body, where the pain is, is not necessarily where the problem or solution is.

Chapter Two

Toes Forward

In a full-length leg stride, it is imperative to have your toes pointed forward the whole time! It is easy to think you are doing this when your leg is in front of you. But what people miss, is the technique when your leg is behind you. When your leg is behind you it is easy to turn your foot outwards. In my office I estimate about 80% of people will point their toes outwards and the other 20% will point their toes inwards.

Walking with your toes pointed inwards may lead to pains on the inside of the legs or front of the hips.

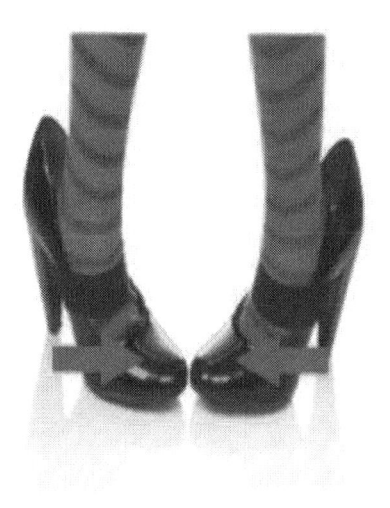

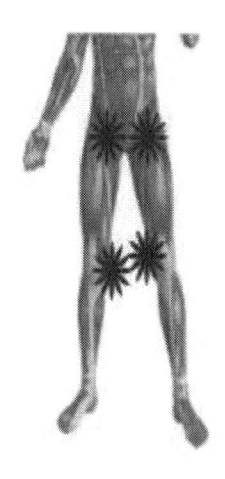

If you walk with your toes pointed outward, you will be using more of the outside leg muscles. Like in Chapter 1, it is key to achieve full range of motion in all joints. If you are only using one side of your leg, this is where shin splints, hip issues and low back pain will develop later. Just like how a pendulum swings your legs and joints must do the same. If you swing one way a certain amount of length, then you need to swing the opposite direction in an equal amount. Problems occur in the joint and muscle length if a joint is flexed in one direction only for a period and rarely flexed the opposite direction. To move forward we are constantly flexing one side of the joint and then the other. If your feet are pointed inward or outward while walking straight ahead over a period, you may create a hip pain like sciatica or low back pain in your back or a hip flexor pain in the front of your hip.

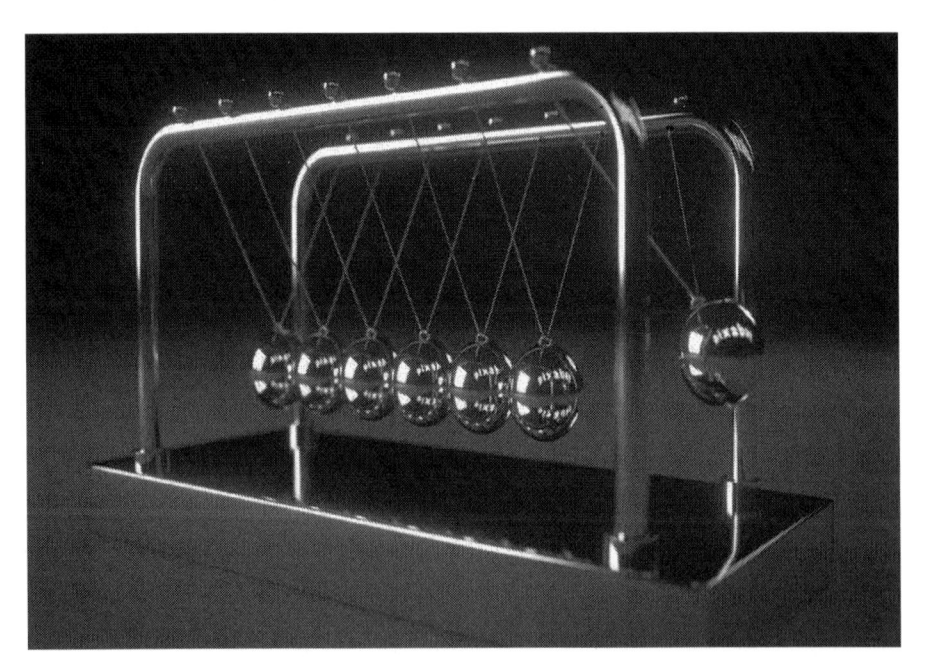

www.pexels.com[1]

The direction of your feet is dictated by your hip muscles when walking. These are referred to as the lateral rotator group. These muscles are called the piriformis, gemellus superior, obturator internus, gemellus inferior, quadratus femoris and the obturator externus. Also, the gluteus group, maximus, medius, and minimus, contributes to pointing the feet out and opening the legs.[2]

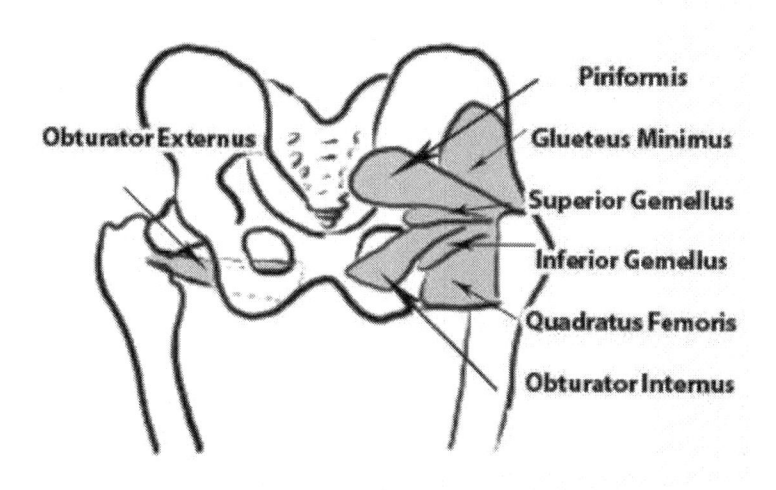

The muscles in the front of your hips, the medial compartment of your thigh, dictate your feet to point inward. The muscles are the gracillis, adductor longus, brevis, and magnus.[3]

When we are walking our lateral and medial hip muscles are what turns our feet. However, when we are in a squatting or sitting position the lower leg muscles will dictate the turning direction of the foot.

When we stand and walk the hip muscles take over the steering of where the body goes.

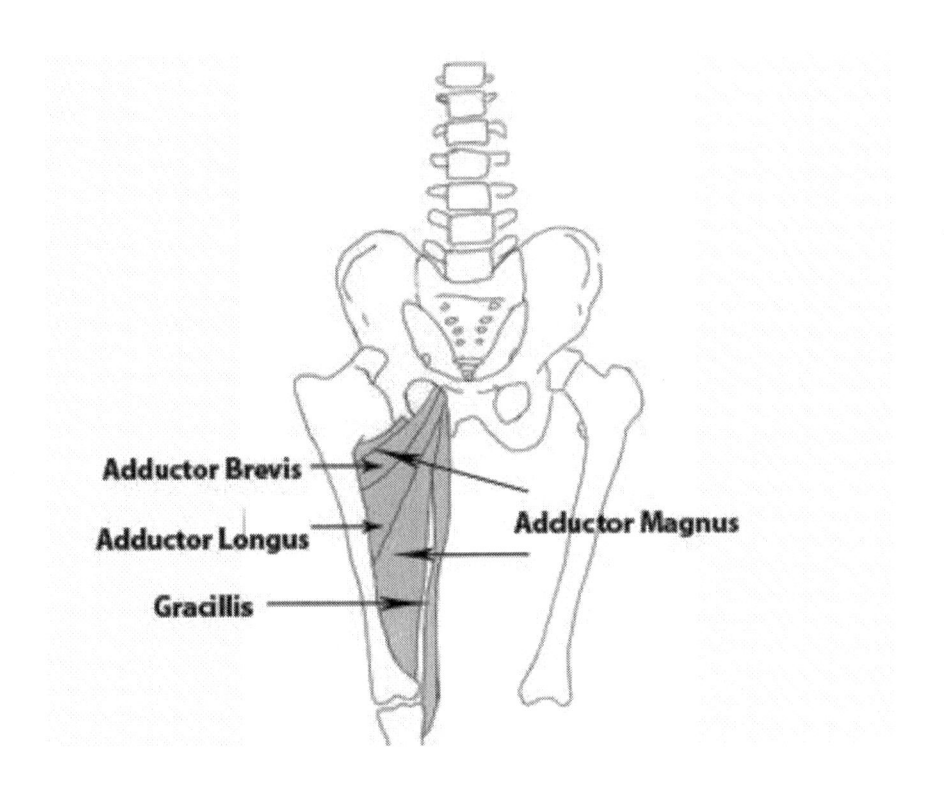

Adductor Brevis

Adductor Longus

Gracillis

Adductor Magnus

Muscle imbalances are thought to be caused by abnormal afferent stimuli due to tension, trauma, poor posture, joint blockage, painful or noxious stimuli, excessive physical demands and habitual movement patterns. Of course, neurologic and genetic factors also play a major role. Some conditions are serious, and others are not.[4]

-Erik Dalton, Ph.D.

Each of these muscle groups has the responsibility of taking an appendage one way and the opposing group takes the appendage the other way. Both are working toward a common goal of equally sharing the work of moving the appendage one way and then the other direction. Problems will occur when one group is constantly doing more work than the other. When we are out of balance or have improper posture, our joints will not line up properly. This will lead to muscles fatiguing faster than usual. When a muscle is overworked or fatigued, it tightens up and shortens in length. When a muscle is shortened it will pull the joint out of place and it will stay out of place. The joint will begin to harden because it is not in the correct posture, so it will protect itself by hardening. In between these tight muscles runs nerves. When these muscles are shortened and tight they lose their pliability and become hard. If these muscles are forced to do a

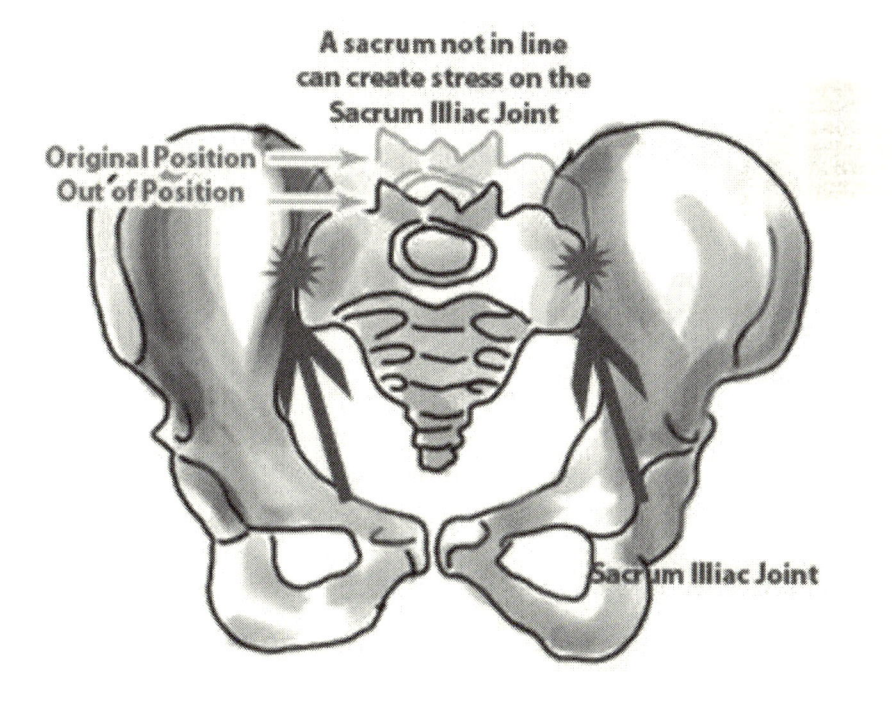

A sacrum not in line can create stress on the Sacrum Illiac Joint

Original Position
Out of Position

Sacrum Illiac Joint

different activity going in another direction or forced, like a whiplash in a fall or car accident, they will be stretched and the nerve between them will be squeezed, pinched, or pulled. This is usually the case with a tendonitis or nerve inflammation pain. If the muscle is damaged it will swell and a "ballooning" effect will push on the nerve.

In the case of the hips, a common issue is sciatica. Sciatica is referred to the sciatic nerve is being compressed in some way. It can be due to a misalignment of the lower vertebrae discs or sacrum being herniated. If the muscles in the lateral rotator group are tight, specifically the piriformis muscle, it can squeeze or stretch the sciatic nerve causing pain to travel down the leg. This issue can also be referred to as the piriformis syndrome.[5]

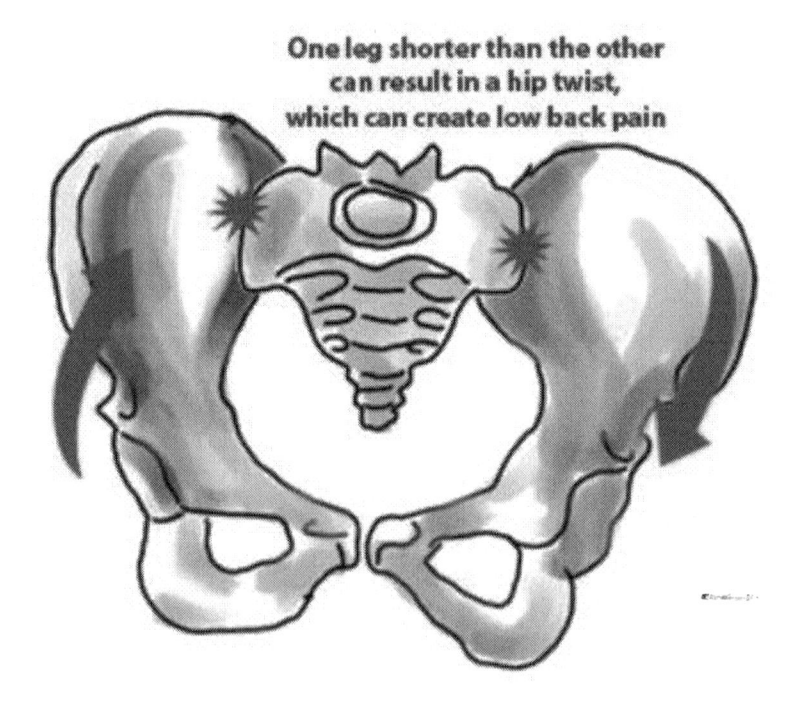

One leg shorter than the other can result in a hip twist, which can create low back pain

The Sacral Iliac Joint (SI Joint) can also be affected by a misalignment of muscles due to walking with your feet pointed inwards or outwards.

The sacrum is a nexus of nerves that radiates from the center of the tailbone and travel down through the legs. If there is a misalignment of the sacrum, hip bone, or hip joint this can also be a chronic issue.

All these issues can be pinpointed to an imbalance of the internal and external muscle groups not sharing an equal load of the body. One of the main purposes of these muscle groups is about turning your feet in or out. Regarding Walking naturally these muscles assist with making

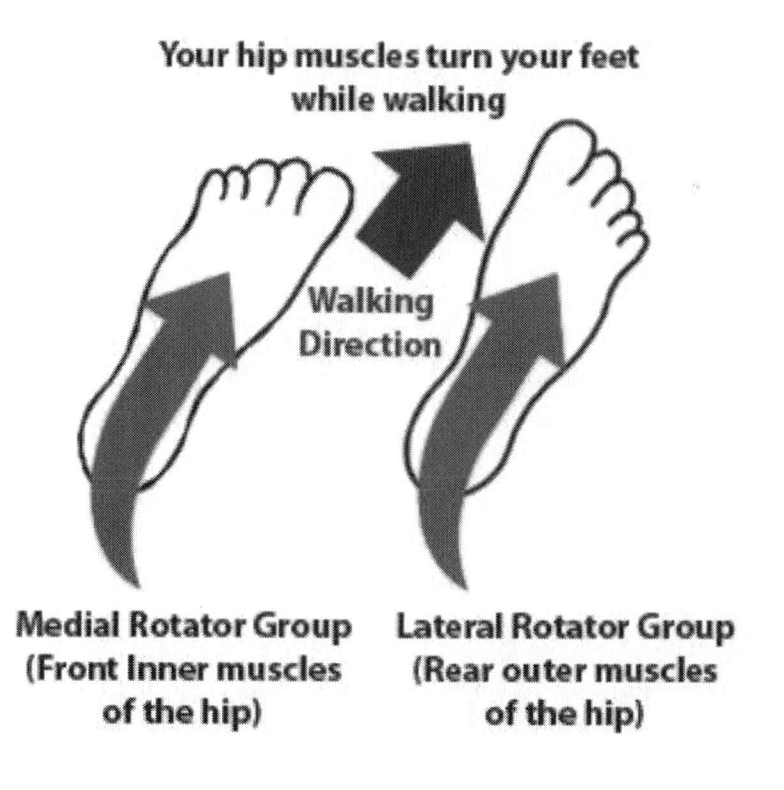

Your hip muscles turn your feet while walking

Walking Direction

Medial Rotator Group (Front Inner muscles of the hip)   **Lateral Rotator Group (Rear outer muscles of the hip)**

turns while you walk. When you are walking, and you are going to turn right, you will use your rear external rotating muscles to turn your right foot outward. Your left leg is going to use the internal rotating muscles to turn your leg and foot inward. This is how you will turn right and vice versa for turning left. You are using both muscle groups. However, a lot of people when walking straight ahead will have their feet pointed outward or inward. Your feet should be pointed straight ahead when going straight. Problems occur if you do things like have your feet continually pointed outward. This means you are continually flexing your lateral rotator muscles and not ever countering these muscles by using your internal rotators. If you are using turning muscles while walking straight ahead, you could be straining and squeezing your SI Joint and/or your hip/leg joint out of place creating a lot of these issues like bursitis, sciatica, and low back pain.

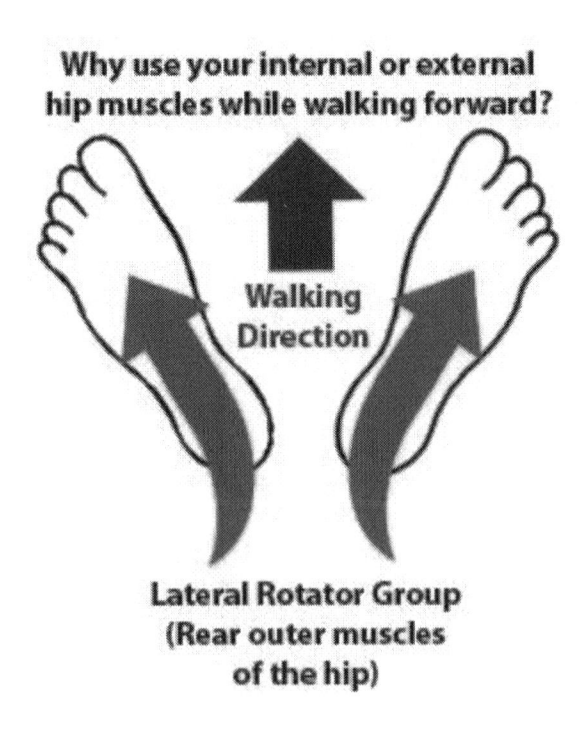

Why use your internal or external hip muscles while walking forward?

Walking Direction

**Lateral Rotator Group
(Rear outer muscles
of the hip)**

When you are walking forward you should NOT be using the medial (internal) or lateral (external) muscles groups. They should be relatively relaxed as they are just for turning. However, if your feet are not pointed straight ahead you will be using these muscles. When you use a muscle group that is not intended for that motion then the joint will slowly be pulled out of position. When muscles and joints are not in the correct position they will harden and then one mis-step and they will break like glass. This will later cause inflammation and then progress to a more constant chronic issue. If you continually walk this way you will be creating a constant inflammation response and the muscle or joint will not heal. When you flex the muscle into the correct position your body will go towards healing.

When we turn our legs in or out we are moving the position of the joint itself. So, if we are intending to walk straight ahead but we are using muscles that turn our leg in or out, we are compromising the muscles that move our legs forward. If we turn the wheels of a car outward and then demand it go straight ahead, there will be some strange sounds from the wheels and axle. This may be a more dramatic example to a

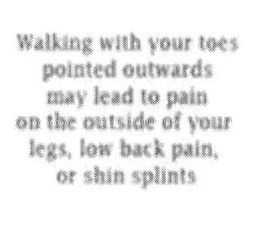

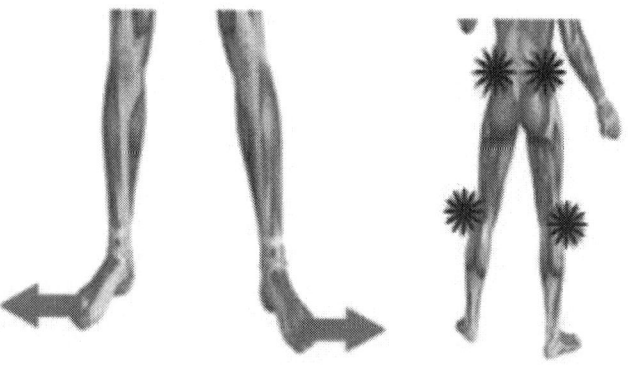

Walking with your toes pointed outwards may lead to pain on the outside of your legs, low back pain, or shin splints

hip misalignment, but over time this will stress the hip joint and break a car.

To walk forward we use bigger and stronger muscles. To move our leg forward we use our front thigh muscles to extend our lower leg forward. Some of these hip muscles are the psoas and iliacus. When our leg is behind us we use our gluteus and hamstrings to move our thighs backwards. All these muscles are large and strong. So, when we have our legs turned inward or outward as we are walking straight ahead, we are misaligning our hip joint which strains the hip rotators and does not allow the full strength of motion for these large muscles to do their primary job.

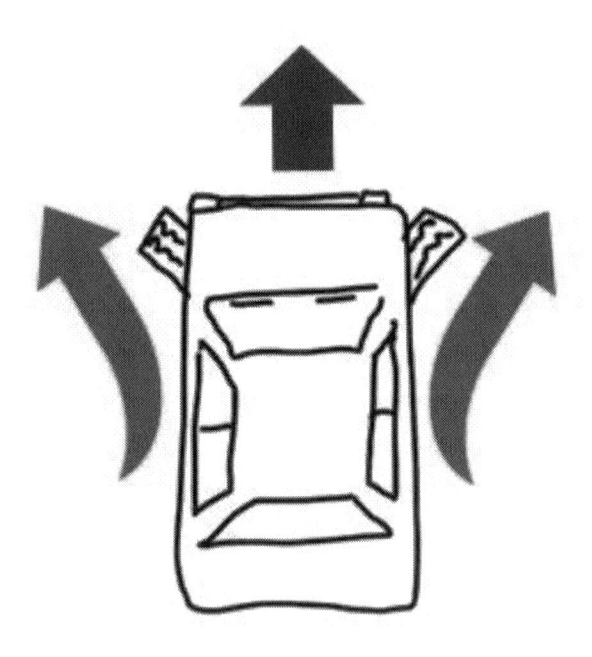

When toes are pointed in or out you will fall over

For a moment, try standing with your toes pointed outward and keep your back straight. You may notice that you begin to fall backwards. To keep from falling backwards one must slightly curve their spine and head forward to counter the balance. People who walk or stand with their toes pointed outward will often report neck and mid-back pain due to stress on their spine.[6]

When the toes are pointed forward for the whole leg stride, this will move the chest back and your head will go backwards. Then your spine will align correctly, and your head will rest on top of your cervical spine.[7]

Toes Pointed Outwards

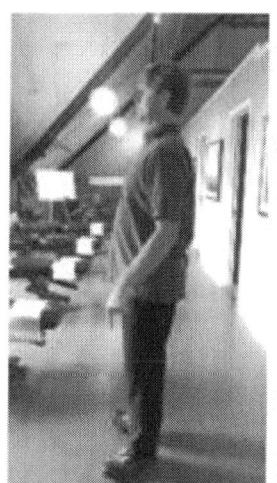

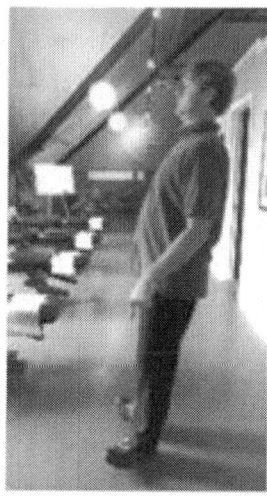

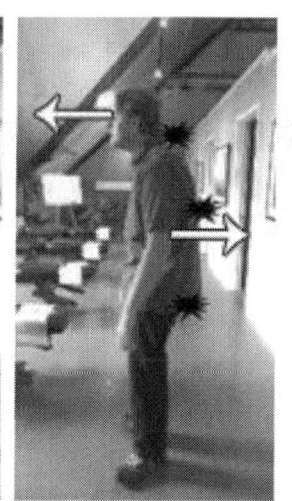

When toes are pointed outwards people will fall backwards.

This is the posture people will be in to keep from falling over.

Posture of people who walk with their toes pointed inward (overpronation and falling arches)

When people walk with their toes pointed inward, they will start to fall forward. Like the exercise before keeping your back straight and point your toes inward. Observe how your center of weight moves forward and then you begin to fall forward.

Inward toe walkers may have tightness in front of the hips, thighs, and front of the calves from this incorrect walking technique. Since they

Toes Pointed Inwards

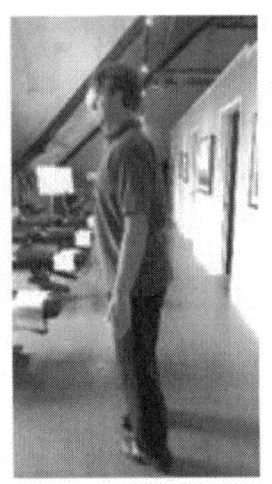

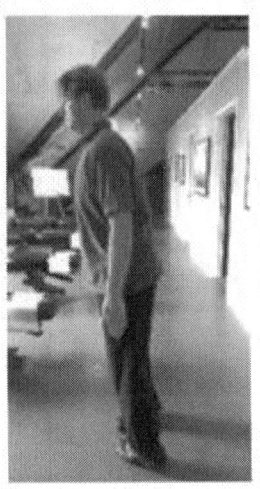

When toes are pointed inwards people will fall forward.

This is the posture people will be in to keep from falling over.

are continually falling forward they may over arch their back which will tilt their hips forward causing low and mid back pain.

Inward toe walkers may also fall into the category of overpronation. This is where people's weight is falling inwards. Falling arches is an issue that can be created here as well.[8] In the Chapter of "No more falling arches", this information will help correct these issues.

Toes inward or outward can create Knee Pain

A secondary issue that can be created by walking with your toes pointed inward or outward is knee and ankle pain. When you are working one muscle group more than it's opposing muscle group, the group that is working more will become tighter and shorter and the opposing muscle group working less will become longer. For instance, those that walk with their toes pointed outward will be walking on the outside's edges of their feet. The outside leg muscle groups are the IT

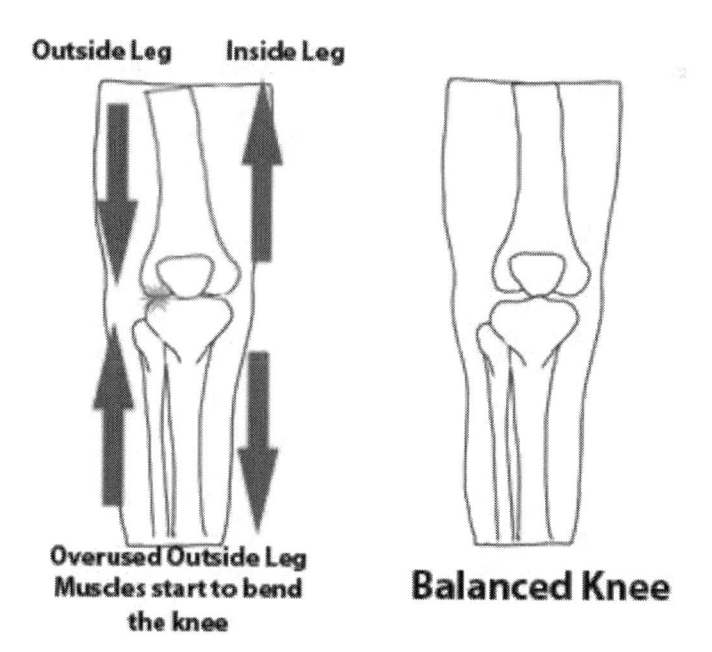

Outside Leg   Inside Leg

Overused Outside Leg Muscles start to bend the knee

Balanced Knee

band, outer shin muscles. This will shorten the outside leg muscle and lengthen the inside leg muscles. The knee will be in the middle and will slightly bow inward. The knee joint will be misaligned creating the cartilage between the knees to be closer together which will create less cushion tolerance for impacts. The MCL and ACL ligaments that support the integrity of the knee will also be misaligned. When misalignment happens, these soft tissues will harden and if under stress they will break easier. This may also lead to ACL and MCL sprains and tears to happen easier because the pliability has been lessened.

If one has already torn one of these ligaments it is important in rehabilitation to make sure you are walking straight ahead to strengthen these muscles. After we are injured we tend to walk on the uninjured leg more, which further compromises the joint and may prolong recovery. After the inflammation and tenderness of an injury is gone it is important to strengthen the surrounding muscles in the correct alignment.

In conclusion, when walking, having your toes pointed forward will help in preventing and alleviating leg and hip pain. If there is a problem with the hips you may want to look down, because some of the problems will be the positioning of your feet.

In the next Chapter "The Four Step Points", it will be imperative to have your toes pointed forward or you will find it very difficult to hit all 4 Step Points. By the end of the Chapter there is a list of issues that may be created if you miss any of the 4 Step Points. Straight ahead we go…

Chapter Three

The 4 Step Points

Now we get a little more detailed and break up the foot into 4 specific contact Stepping Points.

Step Point 1: Heel

Step Point 2: Outside Ball of Foot

Step Point 3: Inside Ball of Foot

Step Point 4: Big Toe

26

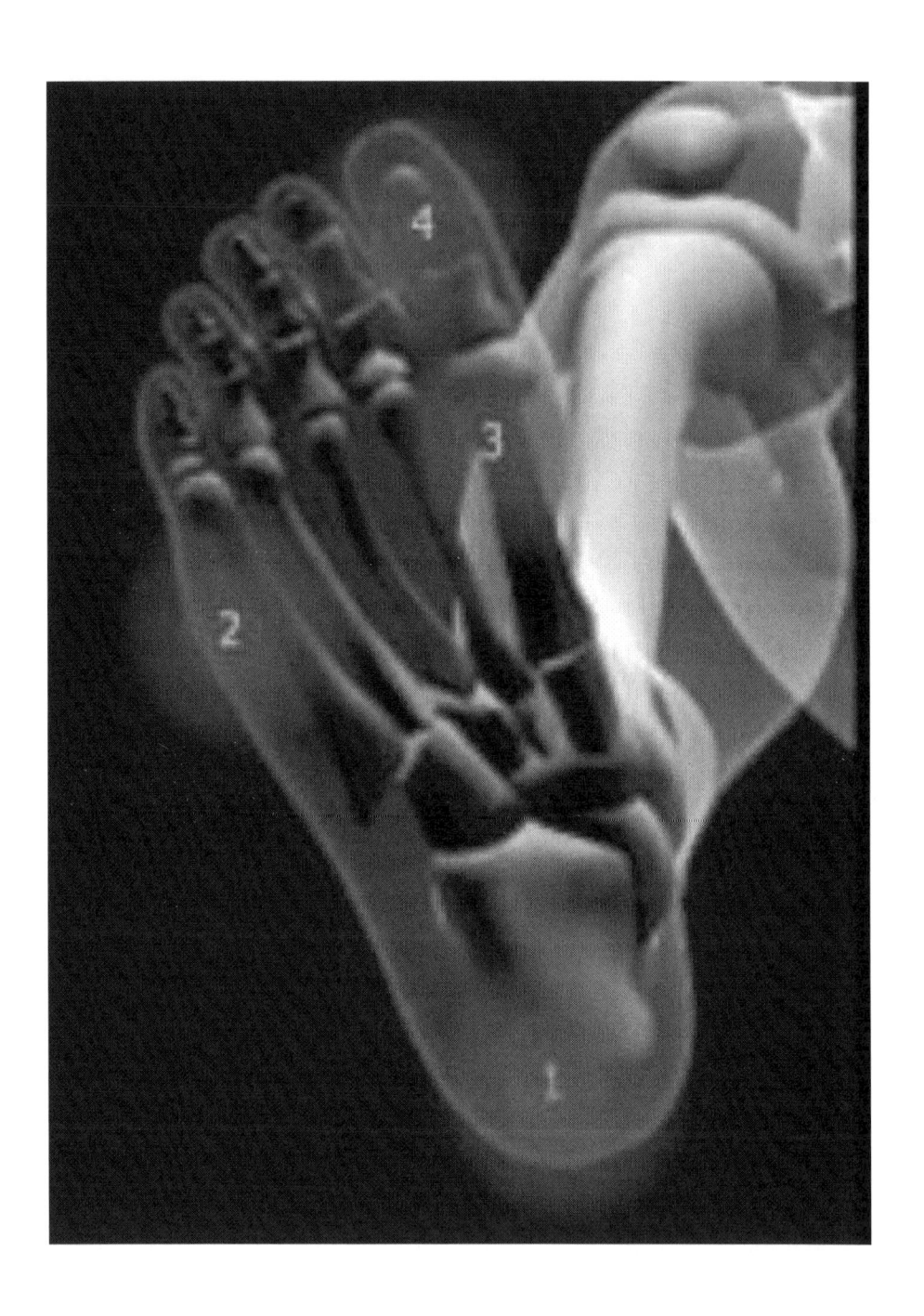

It is important to hit each point individually. One point will lead into the next one. So if a Step Point is not hit firmly it will accumulate into bigger problems later. Each Step Point activates a certain muscle group that supports a specific posture balance. How the feet engage the ground will be the foundation for the rest of your body.

Walking and posture is a lot like learning math. First we start out with adding and subtracting. Every year we learn a new math lesson that builds upon the last. If we skip any of these lessons it will become nearly impossible to understand advanced math.

This same accumlation of lessons is just like learning to walk. If we do not understand these Four Steps Points and skip some of them, it will be a lot like never learing to add. As we move up the body an anccumulation of pain can radiate up the body. Most body posture pain can be pin-pointed to not engaging one of the Four Step Points.

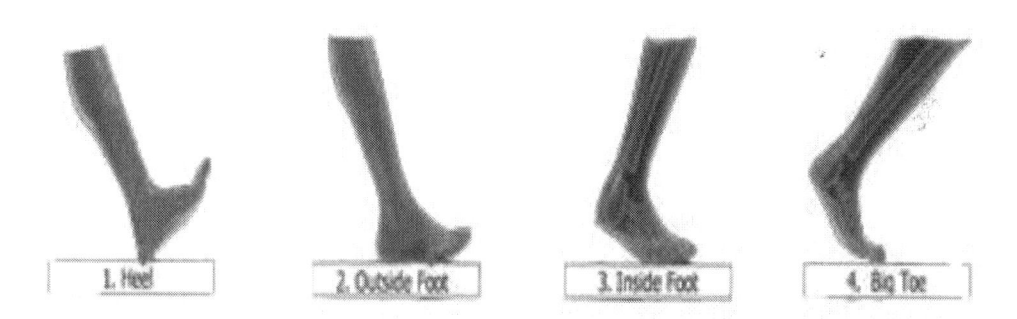

1. Heel	2. Outside Foot	3. Inside Foot	4. Big Toe

Alternating between Outside and Inside Leg Muscles

It is important to hit Step Point 1 and 2 when your leg is in front of you. Step Point 3 and 4 occur when your leg is behind you.

Also, take notice of the muscles in your legs while you're walking. When your leg is in front of you, you will use the outside and front leg muscles. When your leg is behind you, you are going to use your inside and rear leg muscles.

While you are walking, your feet should behave like a wave fluctuating from outside to inside, while rocking back and forth. However, to the observer, it will look like nothing is going on.

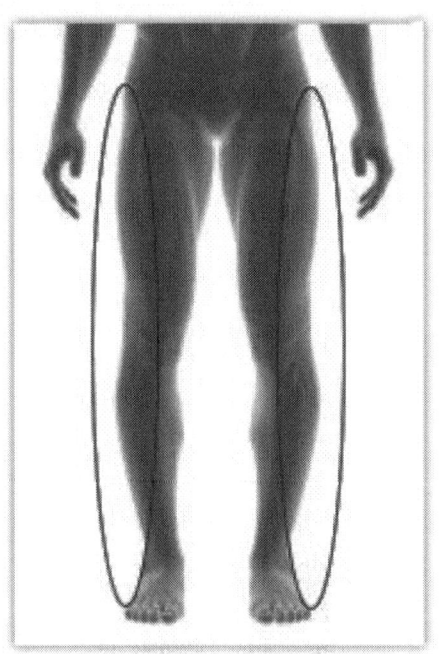

Outside Leg Muscles 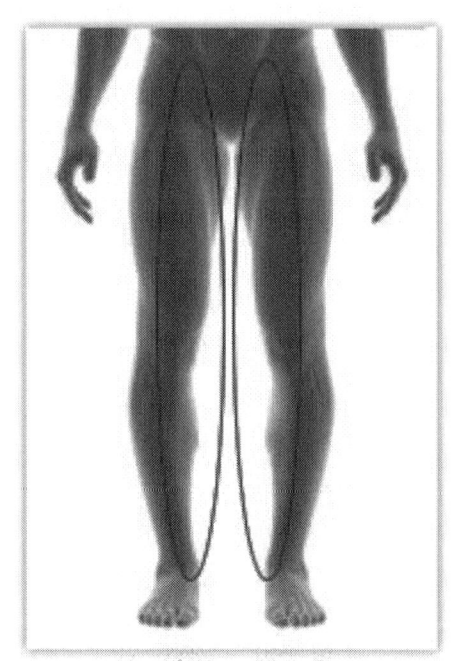 · Inside Leg Muscles

Skipping any of these points may create a variety of commonly known issues

Skipping Step Point 1, like discussed in Chapter One, may create achilles tendonitis. Not lifting your foot up enough will not stretch out the achilles. Those who walk like this tend to have their weight centered on the back of their foot which will harden the achilles. Those that have ruptured an achilles likely have missed this detail for a long time.

A secondary detail is to square up the foot when your heel is about to hit the ground. If your outside heel of your shoe is worn away it is likely you are hitting your heel and foot to the ground at an angle. If you do walk like this, you will predominantly be using Step Points 1 and 2. Due to the angle of your foot it will be very difficult to really flex the inside foot which is Step Point 3 and 4. This is likely to create pains like low

Squaring your Foot before your heel hits the ground

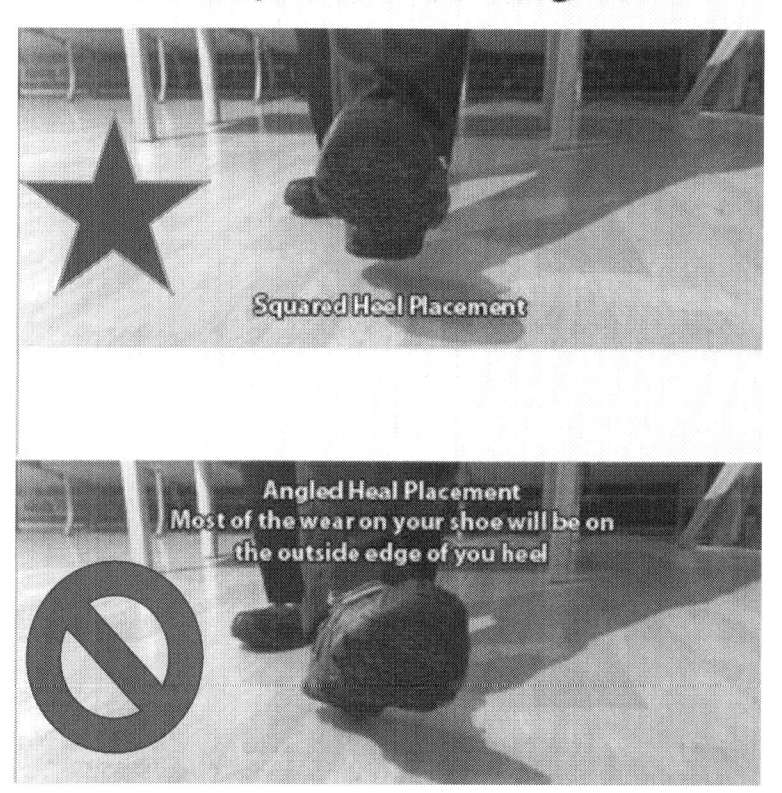

Squared Heel Placement

Angled Heal Placement
Most of the wear on your shoe will be on the outside edge of you heel

back pain and sciatica. People who have injured their toes are likely to walk this way also.

Those that skip Step Point 2 may overpronate. Stepping first on the inside of one's feet may lead to falling arches and plantar fasciitis symptoms. If one does not flex the arch of the foot the arch will fall. This is often what arch support companies are selling to people who do this. If you flex your arch you will prevent these issues and may likely not need arch supports. See Chapter "Gripping the Ground, No More Falling Arches".

Shin Splint Resolution

Skipping Step Point 3 may lead to shin splints. Often these people are heavy on Step Points 1 and 2 and don't move their weight over to Step Point 3 and 4. By just using the outside leg muscles more than the inside leg muscles may result into shin splint creation.

As previously mentioned with squaring up the foot, shin splint creators are likely not doing this as well. Shin Splints is due to pinching the nerves inside the lower leg.[1] If one is predominantly using Step Points 1 & 2 then the outside leg will be tight (short) and the inside leg will be overstretched (long). The outside leg muscles are extensor hallucis, extensor digitorum longus, fibularis longus. The inside leg muscles are the flexor digitorum longus and flexor hallucis longus. These muscles help angle the foot in the side to side axis plane (See 3 Axis's Chapter). When the foot is always at an angle then the muscles will not line up correctly and will inflame[2]. This inflammation will squeeze the nerves inside the lower leg, thus shin splints[3].

How to resolve shin splint pain is to strengthen the inside leg muscles. I had crippling shin splints when I was playing softball. I was a competitive swimmer, so we did not do much running. So, when it came to the running sports my legs seized up quickly and walking to my car after a game was very difficult. This event is what inspired me to right this book because by the next season I had totally overcame my shin splint pain and I have never had them again.

I started to flex my inside legs and would only walk on them. (Of course, you need to look around first to make sure no one is looking because this will look odd to any observer). Much like how a skater uses their inside leg muscles to move forward. I walked the same way down the sidewalk. I would press off the inside leg muscles slaloming back and forth. This aligned my lower leg muscles.

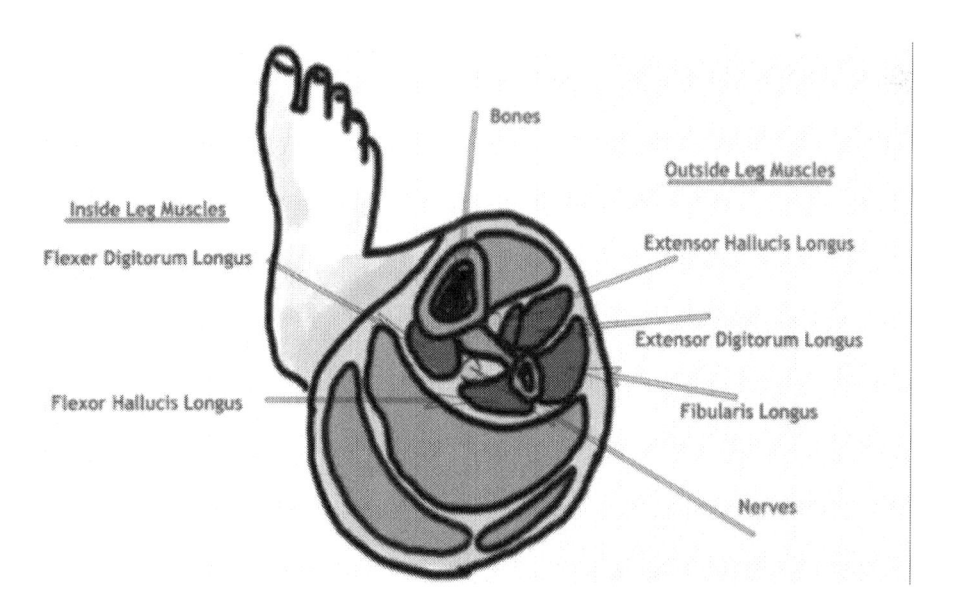

Bones

Outside Leg Muscles

Inside Leg Muscles

Flexer Digitorum Longus

Extensor Hallucis Longus

Extensor Digitorum Longus

Flexor Hallucis Longus

Fibularis Longus

Nerves

Outdoor and Indoor Skating

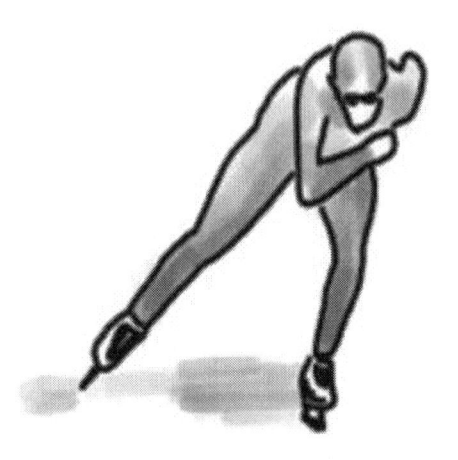

Inside leg muscles will help resolve shin splints,

which is the same motion as skating

Pain is because muscles are flexed out of place. We must flex them back into place. There are a lot of stretches out there for shin splints. But you cannot stretch a muscle back into place, it must be flexed. The StretchFlex Chapter will go into more detail on why.

So, when looking at the "square your feet" picture and the foot is landing on the outside edge. To relieve shin splints your want to do the opposite and over flex your inside foot and push off it just like a skater.

Low Back Pain and Sciatica Resolution

It's estimated that up to 80 percent of adults experience persistent symptoms of lower back pain at some point in their lives. 31 million Americans struggle with the condition at any given time. Given its extremely high prevalence rate, whether due to a weak psoas muscle, sciatic nerve pain or some other cause, it's not surprising that lower back pain is considered the single leading cause of disability worldwide according to the American Chiropractic Association, with half of all American workers reporting having occasional back troubles each year.[4]

Skipping Step Point 4 is one of the main contributors to low back pain. It is done by not having your feet pointed straight ahead. People are not pushing off their big toe and staying more on the outside leg muscles. This means your feet are really pointed outwards and this will create symptoms like low back pain and sciatica. I have seen this a few times with people who have broken their big toe. This however, creates low back pain and some cases neck pain because of the way the angle of the foot hits the ground.[5] This will lead the person to lean more on the outside leg muscles of the leg with the broken toe. The more one leans to one side, the more the head will be off-center. I have seen a few times that if someone has broken their right big toe they will have left chronic neck pain. When you are off balance with your feet your head will have to counter the body imbalance, otherwise you will fall over.

Again, the squaring of the foot to the ground is important. If your foot is hitting the ground at an angle it will be very difficult to then push off Step Points 3 and 4. Step Point 3 and 4 must be hit separately![6]

When you hit them separately that means your foot is forward the whole stride. Usually people are hitting Step Point 3 & 4 at the same time and then their foot is at an angle throughout the whole stride. So now this person will only be using their outside leg muscles and their hips will fall backwards which may create low back issues. By straightening out your foot and hitting Step Point 3 and 4 **separately** you will be engaging your inside legs, which will correct your hip alignment. Now you will begin to resolve your low back issues.[7]

Plantar Fasciitis

Skipping Step Points 1 and 4 is how to create plantar fasciitis. These people are not lifting their foot enough before the heel hits the ground and are also not pushing off the ground enough when their foot is behind them.[8] Walking is a lot like catching and throwing a ball. When we are walking we are opening our foot to catch the ground, so then we can throw it. When catching a ball, we want our hand facing the ball, so we can have a better chance at catching it. Then when throwing the ball, we want to square up our hand in the direction we want to throw it for the best accuracy. This is the same thing that needs to happen when walking and aligning our feet and legs. We are catching and throwing the ground with our foot.

If one measured their walking stride one would notice that their overall walking stride is short. Therefore, the full range of motion of the foot opening and closing will not be possible. Then the abductor hallucis muscle is not being flexed or stretched so it will harden. Those that have injured a part of their leg somewhere else is susceptible to this condition. When we injure any part of our leg our body will constrict the movement of the ankle and the opening and closing of the foot to protect the injury. It is important after the inflammation of a leg injury has healed, that we rehabilitate the full range of motion of the abductor hallucis.[9]

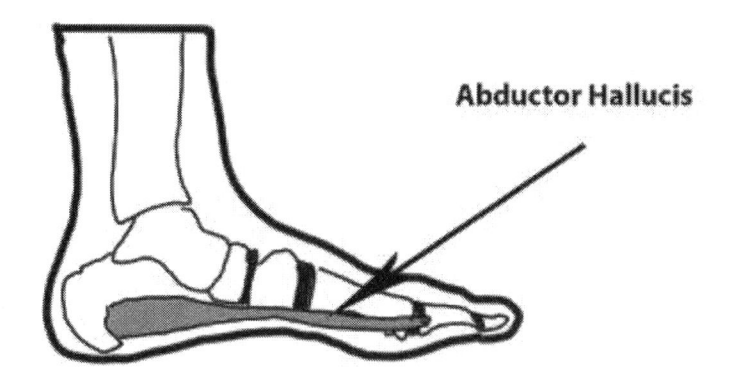

Abductor Hallucis

Chapter Four

Grip the Ground – No more Falling Arches

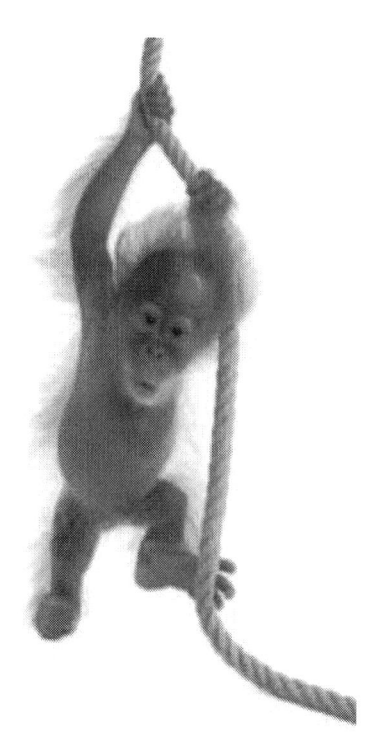

To keep the integrity of your arch, it is a requirement that you have good dexterity in your feet. Gripping the ground and resisting the pull of gravity is important. Arch means bridge, if you do not enforce and maintain the bridge it will fall.

Between the Step Points 2 & 3 is when you transition your outside foot to the inside foot. At this point is where you want to grip and squeeze the ground and feel yourself holding your body up. Falling arches are due to a flaccid foot technique which allows your small bones in your arch to sink down[1]. Strong feet will have strong arches. Plantar fasciitis and falling arches can be prevented here. When practiced properly, this gripping and flexing technique can prevent extreme debilitating pain from occurring. With a little foot flexing, many of your foot pain issues will go away.

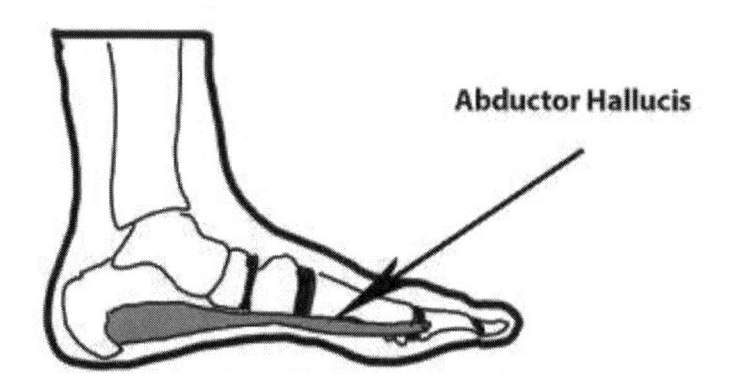

Abductor Hallucis

To prevent falling arches you want to squeeze the abductor hallucis[1] muscle when your foot is directly under your body when walking. It requires one to hit Step Point 3. As you do this you are squeezing together Step Point 3 and Step Point 1 (the heel).

Those that are overpronating, are allowing their arch to fall inward and possibly buckling your knees. Some people will have front hip flexor pain because of this.

High Arches – Flat Feet

Often people are diagnosed with flat feet if they have falling arches and then there are people who have high arches.[2]

Both can have arch pain; however, both are really from not flexing your plantar muscle and letting your arches fall. There are those that diagnose both issues as deformity or genetics, but again I believe it is really a foot flexing technique.[3]

There are those that are born with one leg shorter than the other and some whose joints and bones did not fully develop. According to Dr Joel Wallach this was due to a lack of nutrients from the mother that did not have all the nutrients for the fetus to develop evenly.[4]

Maintaining the Bridge (Arch)

Just like a bridge that is made of stone, so too must your arch maintain its strength and integrity. From the top of the arch to its foundation they must work together, and the bridge will hold.

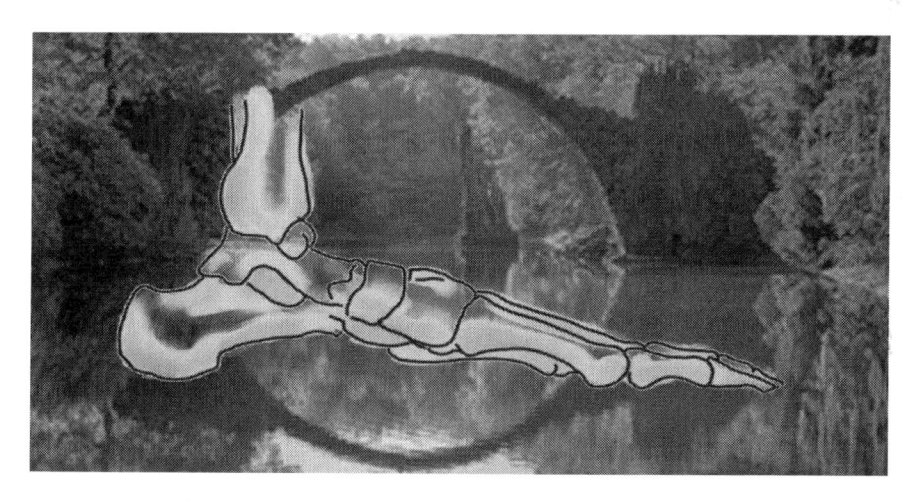

Photo by Martin Damboldt from Pexels [5]

The specific bones of the foot that need to remain in line to prevent falling arches is the Medical Cuneiform and the Navicular.

The Falling Arch

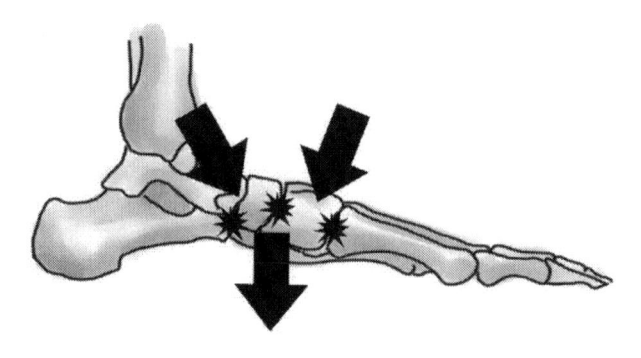

These small bones are positioned at the top of the arch of the foot. If an arch is falling these bones will become misaligned. The integrity of flexing the arch of your foot is paramount in the strength of your foot. Typically, this is where many arch supporting products in shoes are trying to correct for you. It is my opinion that these products are just a band-aid. Sure, they are supporting your arch and keeping it up. However, the flexing of the abductor hallucis is what maintains the arch. The arch of your foot is not just about your foot alone, but it is tied to your overall posture. If you are falling into your arches, then is it very likely your core is not in-shape either thus causing hip and back

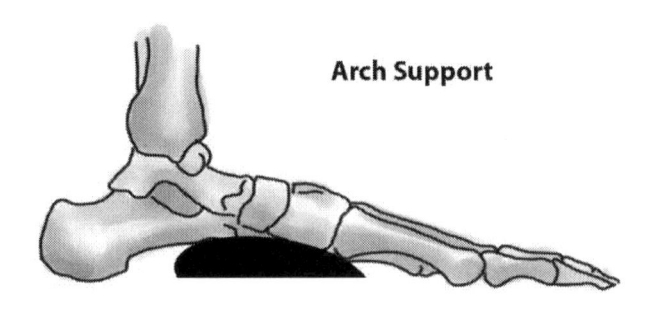

Arch Support

pains. Flexing your arch, with your core (see Core Chapter) will be a big part in contributing to your overall walking posture.

An arch support may get your foot in the right spot; however, the rest of your posture will not be supported. An arch support product will not assist you in flexing your arch. This is like having sand as a foundation to your house. Your house will then be continually sinking, creating other small problems which will turn into bigger and more costly ones later.

"In many cases, abductor hallucis muscle strain is caused by long-standing repetitive microtraumas imposed on the affected structure(s) during the course of normal daily activities especially when one is affected by increased or excessive pronation; as the foot collapses during function due to repetitive inward, downward and forward subluxation (displacement) of the ankle bone upon weight bearing, excessive forces are shifted away from the skeletal structures up to the point one or more soft tissue structures will get overloaded, microtear, inflamed, swollen and tender." [6]

~Ottawa Foot Clinic

The squeezing arch of the foot must be the first technique that needs to be done to cushion your self from the ground. A lot of people say, "running is bad for the legs." [7]

-Dr. David Geier

I don't think running is bad for the legs, but bad technique is bad for the legs. We need to match the pull of gravity on our bodies and stand up straight. The beginning is flexing your arch, and this will help your posture and you'll be able to stand up straight and strong. So much of our pain is because we have a drooping posture due to allowing gravity to pull us down. We need to stand up to gravity and flex our bodies into place. The integrity of the arch will assist in shock absorption as we walk or run. The arch will open and close as we move down the sidewalk. If we do not have this shock absorber our feet will become hard and tight. Then cartilage and joints will be the shock absorber and that is not their main job. One of the functions listed for cartilage is shock absorption, however, heavy long-term shock has been shown to deteriorate cartilage leaving painful conditions like "bone on bone" situations. [8][9]

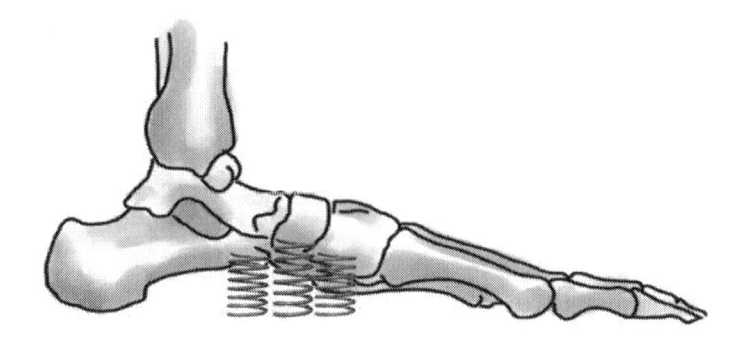

Maintain a spring in your step by toning and flexing your arch.

Tip: The StretchFlex™ Technique for your Arch - step on a tennis ball and roll the ball along your arch while flexing (closing) and stretching (opening) your foot. Suggested time on this exercise is just 2-5 minutes a day. After 1-2 weeks, the pain may be drastically reduced or gone.

Chapter Five

The 3 Axes

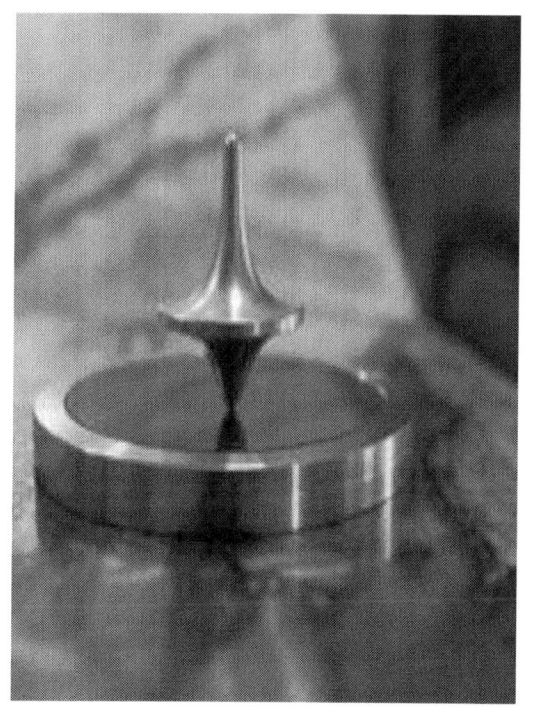

Photo by Ash @ModernAfflatus from Pexels

Now that we have gone over the specifics of foot placement and why it is important to exercise both sides of the joint it's time to put things together. When we are walking our foot needs to bend in 3 different axes'. The 3 Axes' that are foot travels in is up and down, side to side, and open and closed.

Axis 1

In Chapter One, we went over the importance of lifting the foot. This is the first axis, which is about of lifting the foot and then pushing off the foot. This axis is the start and end of the walking stride.

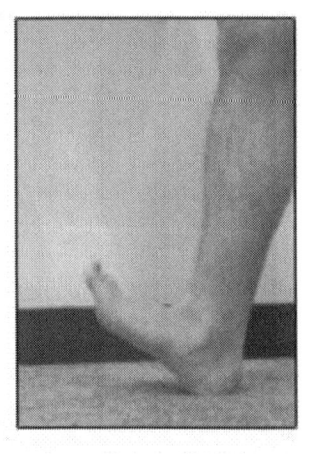

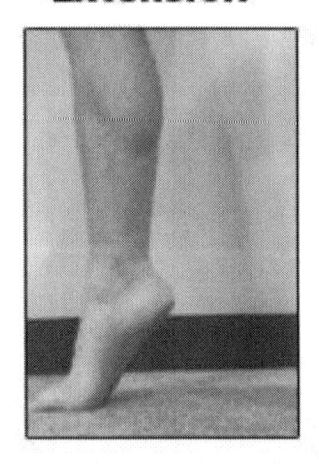

Axis 1

Flexion **Extension**

Axis 2

In Chapter 3 where we get specific with Step Points 2 and 3 which are the inside and outside balls of the feet, we are using the side to side axis. In general, when our leg is in front of us we are using the outside edge of our foot with the support of the outside leg muscles. When our leg is behind us, we shift our weight to the inside edge of our foot using the inside leg muscles for support.

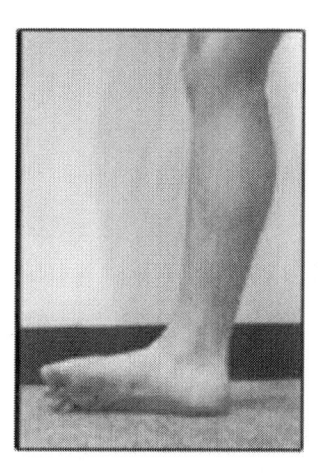

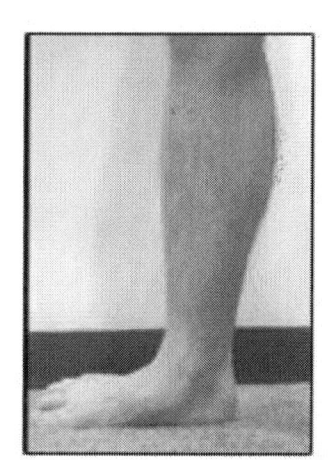

Axis 2

Side to Side

Outside Leg Muscles   **Inside Leg Muscles**

Axis 3

In the "Gripping the Ground" Chapter, we went over the concept of supporting the arch to prevent falling arches. When our heel is about to hit the ground, we open our foot and when our foot is directly below us we are gripping (closing) the ground. So, this axis is used before our heel hits the ground and we open our foot. When our foot is directly underneath us is when we begin to close or grip the ground. Lastly, when we push off our big toe our foot opens again.

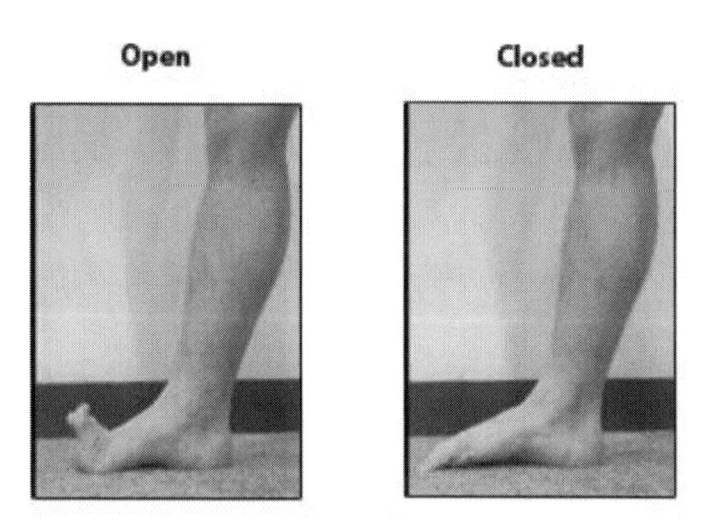

Axis 3

Open **Closed**

So, in total there are 3 axes' that are foot is operating in. It is important to accentuate each axis and when one goes one way we need our foot to go the other way.

There is a fluid motion between each of these axes. Each has a purpose and if we skip one or don't easily transition from one to the next, this is where a pain point can emerge. Walking should be effortless and easy. Focusing on the fine points of how your foot flexes through a stride is important for balance and being pain-free. One misstep here can accumulate stiff muscles further up your body creating sore hips, a spine with scoliosis, or a sore neck creating headaches.

Issues like spinal stenosis could be created by not having a fluid gate. Stenosis is a condition where the vertebrae has osteoporosis. Osteoporosis can be caused due to a compressed spine. If you have very stiff feet you will have an equally stiff hip. Your spine sits on your hips, if you are lacking movement in the axes of your feet, ankles, and your hips, you may be also attributing to the lack of movement in your spine. Not having circulation throughout the body can leave your body in a form of suffocation due to lack of nutrient distribution.[1]

Hips move around like a figure-8

It is important to focus on the finite details of the movement of your feet because your hips will follow what your feet do. It is impossible to have flexible hips if your feet are stiff. The movement of the feet helps accentuate the movement of the hips. If you have a hip problem, it may be very likely you have a foot flexibility issue.

When you are walking your hip is progressing through a figure-8 like movement. When your left leg is moving forward your left hip moves forward. When your leg is beneath you your hip is moving down. When your leg is moving behind you your left hip is moving backwards. Then when your leg swings forward your hip lifts up. Both sides of the hips are moving in constant opposition. When one is up, the other is down. When one side goes forward the other side goes backward.

A lot of sciatic type pain is because the hip is not moving in the full figure-8 motion. If you have low back pain on one side that leg will be shorter, which ultimately means the hip is not moving. Pain happens when there is no movement, things inflame, nerves get squeezed and now you are in a constant chronic condition.

If you have hip issues, look at how stiff your feet are. It is possible your hips have not moved in a long time and you are missing one of the axes'. So, when you are overemphasizing your 3 axes of your feet make sure to allow for your hips to follow the movement. If your hips have been immobile for a long time, it may take a bit to move them again. I suggest going dancing cause you gotta shake it, to make it.

Breathing

When your body has been stuck in the same place for a period there may be some fear around it, especially if it is associated with an injury. Then if you are constantly thinking about technique you may also forget to breathe as well. When we are stressed or stuck in a trauma state your breathing may be shallow.[2]

When we breathe it is important to breathe all the way in and all the way out. Holding your breath will keep your body tight. Full relaxing breaths is like a tranquilizer for your nervous system. When we do an activity like following specific details of your walking gate, we may be holding our breath. Take the moment to overemphasize your breath and your body will loosen up and perhaps your feet will fall in the right position a little easier.[3]

Every time you take a step create a mantra, "that every time I take a step my body becomes looser and more relaxed". Relax into muscles that you have never let go of before. Walking with consciousness, is paying attention to how your body moves. Walking should be effortless and a relaxing activity. I have seen people who have trouble with the concept of walking 4 blocks. Often it is because they have a very tense body, hence why it is such an effort. Holding your breath will keep your body tight. Long slow breaths will help relax the body and if you can do this while walking this will greatly loosen up your body.[4]

Arm Swing

Your arms should swing back and forth if you are walking naturally. There should be little muscle movement in your arms to make them swing. Ultimately your swinging arms are a counter balance to keep you upright. They are correcting your balance as you are walking.

When you move your hips in the figure-8 format your torso will follow and your arms as well. This also helps with the whole walking motion as your arms are then assisting you on swinging your foot forward to take another step.

Having arms that don't swing means your feet are not activating the 3 axes', your hips aren't moving, or you are not breathing. The arms are the last indicator on how well your body is loose and balanced.

Arm and shoulder injuries of the past can affect the arm swing. If they have been injured, then this will affect the balance of how you walk. If one has a frozen shoulder a passive therapy is recommended. Such as leaning forward and let your arm dangle and slightly sway it back and forth. This gets some circulation to the joint. As you are walking let your arms swing and see how much you can let go of the tension in your shoulders.[5]

Chapter Six

Walking Activates Health

"My grandmother started walking five miles a day when she was sixty. She's ninety-seven now, and we don't know where the heck she is."
— *Ellen DeGeneres*

Immune System – Protects the Body

In Acupuncture, the meridian points in the fingers and toes are toning the corresponding organs. In the feet, the Meridians are the spleen, liver, stomach, gall bladder, bladder, and the kidneys. These organs help with overall strength and the immune system. Each of the toning points of organs encircles all areas of the foot, so it is important to tone the muscles of the foot evenly. If a part of the foot is often skipped by lack of circulation and stimulation, that organ may have low energy or restricted flow making the organ "tired" or "sluggish". So, walking naturally and exercising the whole foot will increase overall energy, decrease pain, and promote a stronger immune system.[1]

Lymphatic System – Cleans the Body

In the circulation system, the heart is the muscle that moves the blood throughout the body. In the lymphatic system there is no singular system that moves the water throughout your body. The lymph's are in your arm pits, breasts, sides of the neck, between the legs, and calves. When the surrounding muscles are flexed, this pumps water throughout the body. Walking is one of the best ways to circulate water throughout the body. Where there is circulation, there is healing and strength.[2]

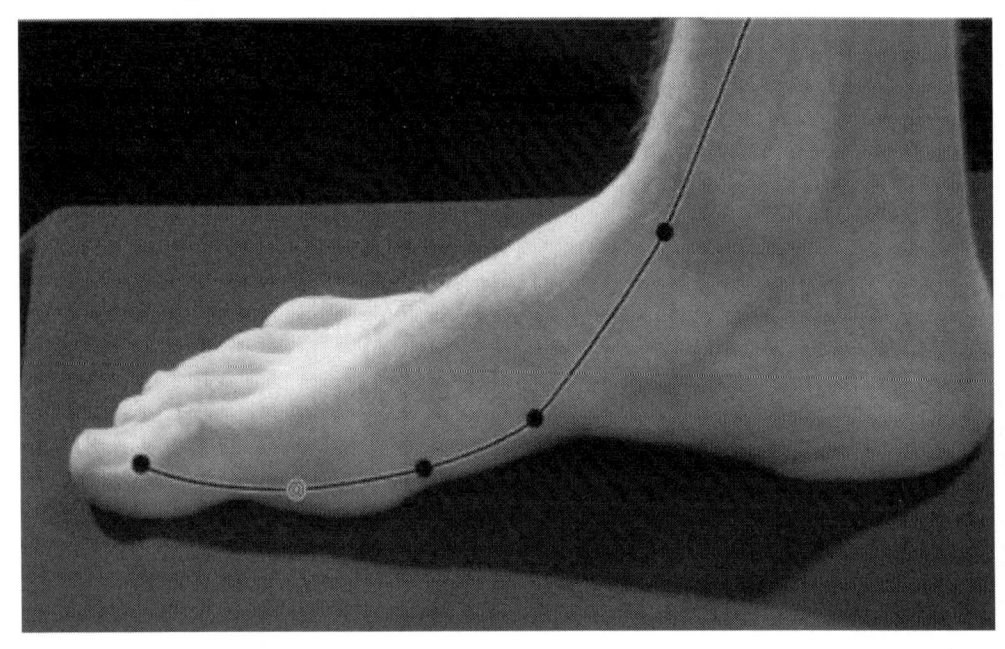

The Path of the Spleen Meridian through the Arch of the Foot (pic. from AcuGraph)

Tip: Massage is also a recommended way to support the lymphatic system. Squeezing muscles helps pump water through tight areas of the body.

Lymphatic Drainage is a gentle massage technique. This technique is very light and does not engage the muscles. Water moves just below the skin and light strokes in a gentle manner can promote water circulation. When we are sick often our necks will be stiff and achy. This may mean that the lymph nodes in our necks are blocked. Dehydration is likely the cause. When we are sick or injured we need more water than usual to help the body wash out pathogens. Most body pain when we are sick is a signal from the lymph nodes. This is the bodies cry for water.[14]

Reflexology Corresponds to the Walking Technique

When one looks at reflexology charts for the hands, feet, and ears, it will refer to the internal organs and other parts of the body.[1] In reference to the Four Step Points there is also a correlation that can be drawn. How we bend and flex our foot may support the rest of our bodies posture and internal health of specific organs.

Our feet are designed to act as earthward antennae, helping us balance and transmitting information to us about the ground we're walking on. (From "You Walk Wrong," New York Magazine, 28 April 2008)[13]

Before the Heel Hits the Ground

In the first Chapter, "Range of Motion of the Toes is equal to the Range of Motion of the Hips", the flexibility at the ankle will determine how much the hips will open up. It so happens in reflexology the ankle has many points that correspond to the waist and hips.

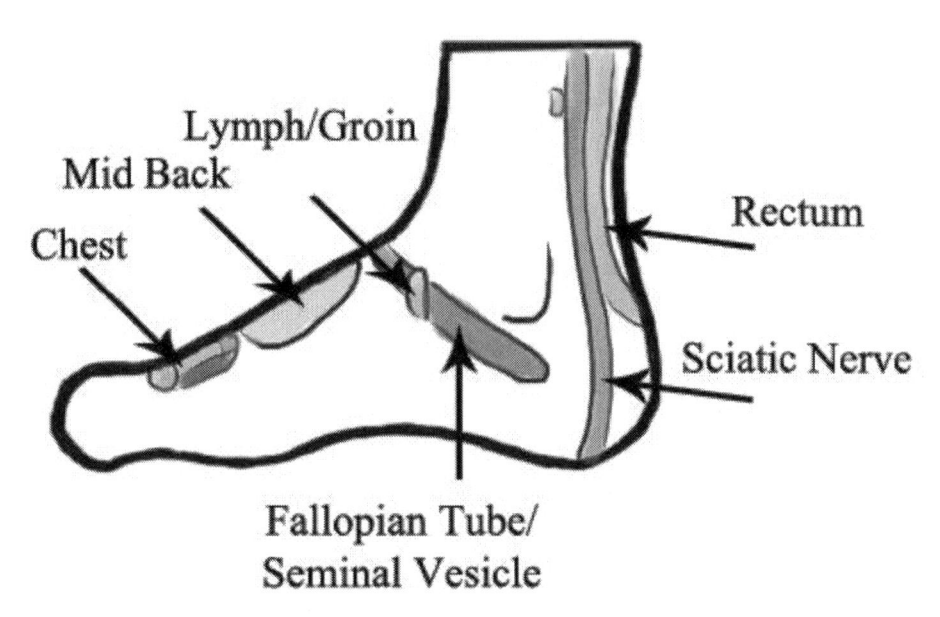

Lymph/Groin
Mid Back
Chest
Rectum
Sciatic Nerve
Fallopian Tube/ Seminal Vesicle

We stress multiple times in this book of opening your foot and lifting it before the heel hits the ground. When we lift our foot, we are bending at the ankle and this stimulates the points in this area. This area in reflexology is the reproduction areas for male and females. The back of the foot in the achilles area is stretched when the foot is lifting and flexing when one pushes off the foot. The achilles area corresponds to the rectum and sciatic nerve. The inside of the heel refers to the uterus and prostate. The outside of the heel refers to the testes, ovaries, and the hip sciatic area. So, the heel refers a lot to the lower areas of the front and back hips and the tailbone including the sciatic nerve.[2]

Before the heel hits the ground, we are opening the foot by lifting the toes and bending up at the ankle. These reflexology points of the toes refer to the front of the chest and the jaw. The top-middle area of the foot refers to the mid-back. When we open and lift our foot this will keep us from falling forward. If we do not activate this part of the foot, people's postures tend to fall forward, and the back will round forward as well. Opening the foot assists in pushing the chest, neck, and shoulders back and therefore the midback will not be rounded forward but will stay in an upright posture. Peoples head usually tends to jet forward, however, when one lifts the toes this will move the head back into a position where the cervical spine is the original supporter.

Try standing on one leg and lift the other leg up in the air, then lift the toes upwards. Notice how that action alone subtlety lifts your body up. Without this action we tend to fall forward, and this simple action will keep us upright and keep one from rounding their back.

The bottom side of the toes refers to the brain, eyes, and ears. So, it is important at the beginning and end of the stride to open and flex the toes as this may assist neck issues and stimulate the senses.[3]

Step Point 1

Now that we have opened our foot we will activate Step Point 1 which is the bottom of the heel. The heel refers to the sciatic nerve, coccyx, and lower sacrum. When our leg comes forward to step on the heel we are stretching the sacrum area. Short walking strides and not lifting your foot may create a limited range of motion for the rear of the hips. When we push off our big toe we will be flexing our rear. So, a full ankle range of motion will assist in maximizing the full range of motion of the sacrum area.

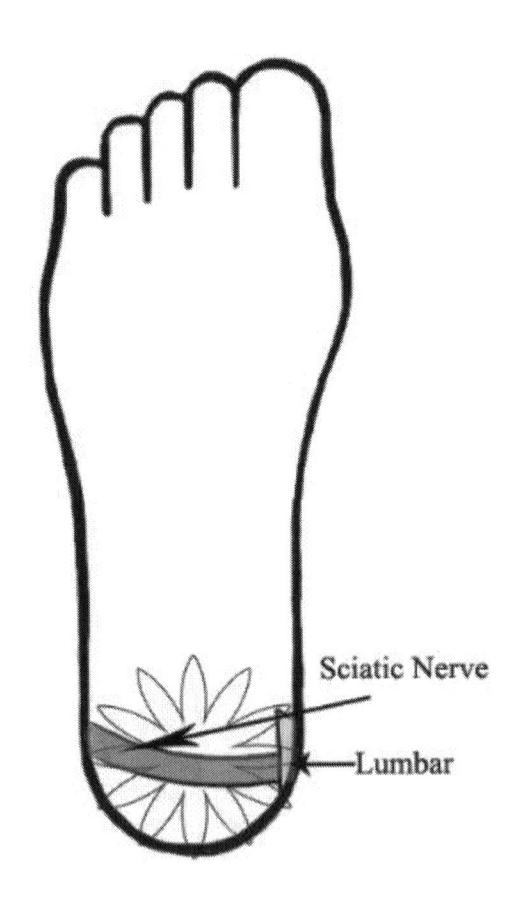

Sciatic Nerve

Lumbar

Step Point 2

Step Point 2 (outside ball of the foot) directly activates the shoulders and arms. The distance between the Step Point 1 (heel) and Step Point 2 is activating the legs and the large and small intestines. Other internal organs are the gall bladder, liver, and spleen located in the outer edges of the foot between the heel and arch.

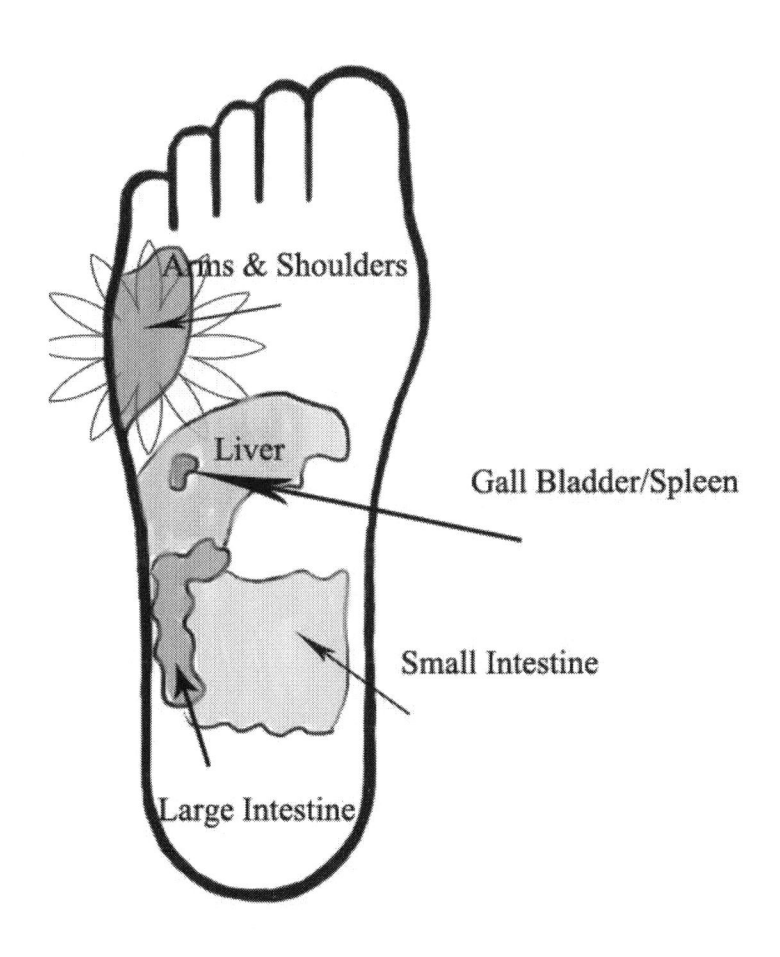

At Step Point 2, the toes are beginning to be flexed, starting with the outside smallest toe and then crescendo's up to the big toe. The flexing of the toes is assisting with shifting of weight from the outside to the inside leg muscles.[4] The points that are activated are mostly inside the head, starting with ears, eyes, sinus's and the brain. In yoga a mantra is "old age starts in the toes". In a lot of older people hearing is one of the senses that is compromised. The inner ear assists with balance and equilibrium. Do people with hearing issues have stiff toes?[5]

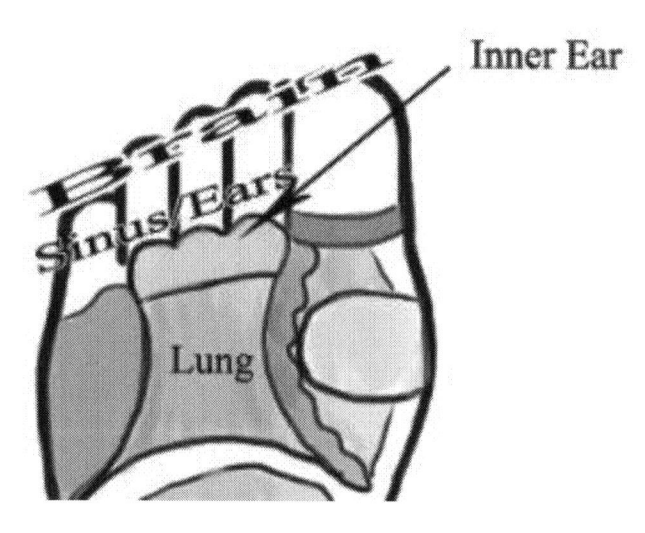

Step Point 3

In the transition between Step Point 2 and 3 a lot of things are activated. Step Point 3 (inside ball of foot) activates the heart, bronchial tubes, thyroid, vocal cords, and the front of the chest. Seems this point is most active with the front of the chest and neck. So, when we use Step Point 2 we activate the back of the shoulders and chest, and then transition to the front of the chest region. The lungs and the diaphragm fall between the middle of the step points in the center of the upper foot, and then finishes with the heart which is Step Point 3. Do people with breathing issues have a stiffness in their gait in this region?

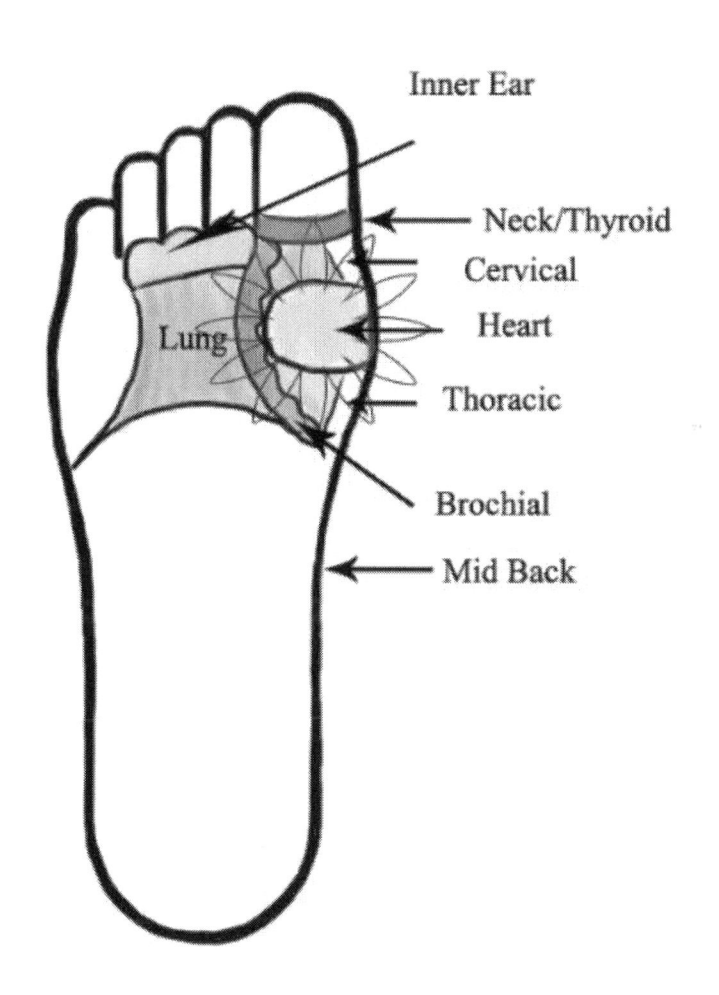

![Foot reflexology diagram showing Lung, Inner Ear, Neck/Thyroid, Cervical, Heart, Thoracic, Brochial, and Mid Back regions]

Step Point's 2 and 3 are about stabilizing the shoulders in the direction of front to back. As we are walking, when we are on these points, our other leg is swinging forward. Our arms are swinging at this time. We are shifting the weight from one leg to the other.[6] If one does not have a noticeable arm swing it may be an indicator that they may not be fully transitioning from Step Point 2 to 3 seamlessly.

The Arch

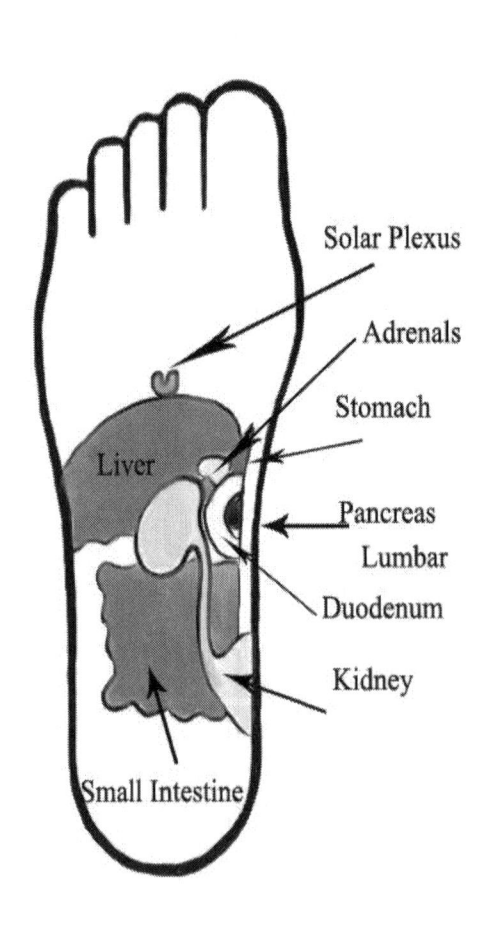

As we make the transition between Step Point 2 and 3 we are starting to activate the foot of the arch. In the arch of the foot, the organs that are stimulated are stomach, pancreas, kidneys, duodenum, solar plexus, and adrenals. These organs are what I call the Strength Chakra in my Medical Intuitive Practice. These organs are about strength and power. As mentioned earlier about the importance to maintaining the arch of the foot, it takes some extra strength to really keep this area in shape. This is the area that connects to our core and connection to the earth. If this area falls or pronates the whole mechanism falls apart.

In a walking stride the gathering of energy is started here. The foot is gripping the ground and using the leverage to later launch the body forward. Kidneys are like the battery packs of the body. Adrenals are the turbo boosts. Pancreas is the fire starter. The core area of the body is activated right here. Think of your arch is the igniter to these organs. The center of your body is balanced by how much one uses the arch of the foot.

When one does not maintain the integrity of their arch and lets it fall, one may be pronating or walking with their toes pointed outwards, both are not using the arch. When one is pronating, the knees can fall inwards and then the body falls forward. When one has their toes pointed outward they will fall backwards. In both cases the core strength and solar plexus of the body is not supported. This will leave the rest of the body to have to make up for the lack of core strength. This may put more stress on the ankles and feet, the hips may have to over flex to assist with the stabilization, and then the neck and shoulders will be in a continuous state of tension due to always being off-centered.[7]

Step Point 4

Step Point 4 is the big toe. Dead center of the big toe corresponds to the pituitary gland, which is the third eye, the decision maker and planner of the way our future will look. In the manifesting process our minds make decisions for our bodies to follow. As our foot has pushed off the big toe it is in the air for a bit. The lift off to the next step, wherever that could be? As this walking step finishes the next step needs to decide what to do next.

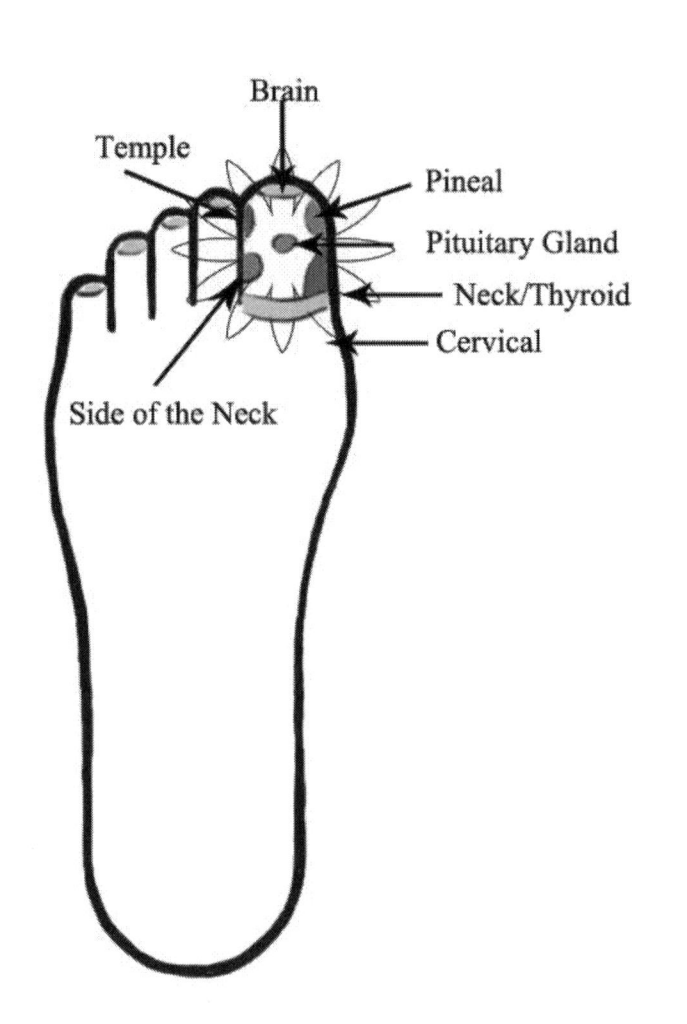

A major item to look at is the "neck" of the big toes which corresponds to the cervical neck.

Previously mentioned is the importance of hitting the big toe separately from Step Point 3. It is important to accentuate the distinction between Step Point 3 and 4 as this is the last fling of the walking stride. At this moment acceleration, deacceleration, or change of direction is the last time things can be changed. The big toe is the last opportunity to correct any movement. If the body is off-centered due to poor posture the neck is going to be the last area to counter balance posture. The flexibility of the big toes can correspond to the flexibility of the neck. When we are flexing the big toe, it may reset our neck into the correct position. Often people's heads are too far forward creating back of the neck pain and headaches. Flexing and pushing off the big toe with full range of motion will send the head backwards if it is too far forward.[9] In my practice I have seen many occasions where one has injured their left toe and will have right neck issues and vice versa.

A study was done with a group of elderly people with leg issues. Practitioners activated the big toe to stimulate the pituitary gland.[11] The pituitary gland secretes growth hormones. Growth hormones help rebuild the tissues of the body including bones.[12] Participants were able to demonstrate improvement to their leg issues.

Spinal Correspondence

The inside edge of the foot corresponds to the whole spine. The wave shape of the inner foot just so happens to curve the same way as the spine. The heel is the lumbar, the arch of the foot is the curve of the low back to the midback and the inside ball of the foot to the big toe is the cervical spine.[8]

So, once again another correlation between the arch of the foot and the low back. Not flexing the arch of the foot will compromise the posture of the midback/low back. When we flex the arch, we are activating inside leg muscles which connects to the front of the hips. Activating the front of the hips positions them in the correct position.

Low back pain can be attributed to a lack of front hip core strength. Flexing your core may alleviate low back pain.

The cervical spine is in the area of Step Point 3 and 4. If these points are not engaged separately the head will fall forward. Flexing these points and pushing off them strongly will reset your head and neck backwards if you tend to fall forward. Falling forward in posture may be due to the lack of rolling off Step Points 3 and 4 separately. So, people who pronate or those that walk with your toe's outwards, both

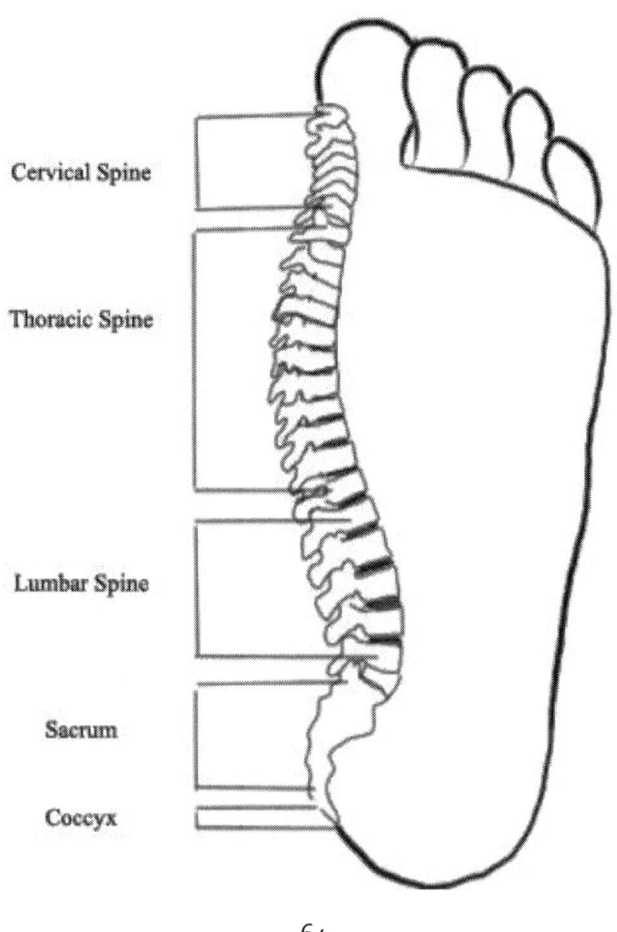

Cervical Spine

Thoracic Spine

Lumbar Spine

Sacrum

Coccyx

groups will not be activating the points that support their cervical spine.

In a walking stride, there is a reoccurring theme that keeps repeating. Starting with the foundation of the body which is the feet and then work your way up. It is important for points and internal systems to seamlessly transition from one area to another. A lack of seamless flow can hinder a walking stride. From heel to toe we are starting at the bottom of the spine and working our way up to the cervical spine. From outside of the legs to the transition of weight to the inside of the legs we are activating points in our body from the back to the front.

Any hitch in this movement can be a beacon that the corresponding point is out of balance and needs some extra attention. Old injuries, potential new injuries, lack of nutrition, depression, low self-esteem, and bad walking habits can all attribute to one missing certain points in their gait. Pain is lack of awareness, let it be your guide in telling you what you need to do, to heal yourself.[10] Be aware of yourself, do you have internal organ issues or chronic pain, does it correspond to your feet and the way you walk?

Chapter Seven

Walking Incorrectly Effects Posture, When one leg is shorter or longer than the other

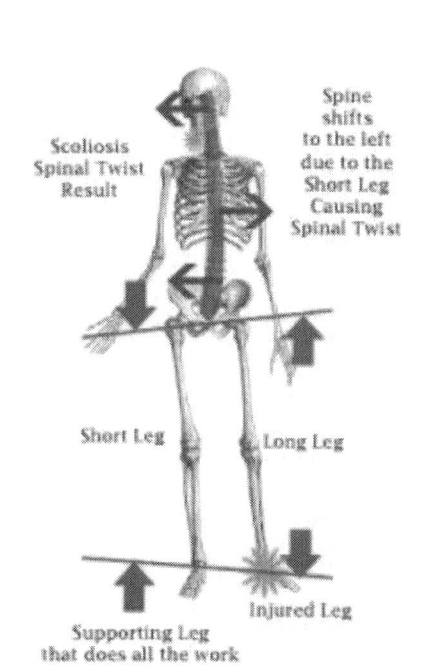

Scoliosis Spinal Twist Result

Spine shifts to the left due to the Short Leg Causing Spinal Twist

Short Leg

Long Leg

Injured Leg

Supporting Leg that does all the work

Walking is something that most people take for granted. In fact, it would never occur to the average person that they might not be walking correctly.

Sciatica occurs because something—bone, disc or muscle—is impinging the sciatic nerve. If we learn to walk and stand correctly, we align our bones in a more effective way, creating a much better pathway for the flow of the sciatic nerve.

- Jonathan FitzGordon

67

Often when one leg is shorter than the other it is because that person leans on the shorter leg more than the other. They do this because in the past they may have sprained or broken something on the opposite leg and they will walk on the healthy leg to relieve pressure on the injured leg. After the injury heals, if they do not walk evenly on both legs, they will continually lean on the "healthy leg".

In some cases, I have seen the opposite posture occur. The short leg will be the injured leg. It depends on when the injury occurred. When the initial injury happens, people will usually shift their weight over the injured leg. After a while, once the initial injury is healed, they may shift their weight to the other leg and lean over that leg. This will start the process again and the person will bounce back and forth with their weight over the leg that hurts less. Even though the healthy uninjured leg is fine it does fatigue quickly due to it doing most of the work of holding up the body. Over time this leg may develop its own cascade of injuries, because you are walking on one leg. The body is meant to walk on both legs evenly. It is important that once the initial injury has healed, that you start working towards equal weight distribution while walking.

If you continually have low back pain on either the left or right side only. Then that is the side that has the shorter leg. It is shorter because when you are injured, your body does not trust it to support the weight of the body. So, the center of your weight shifts over that leg to protect it till it heals. The leg can become shorter by 1/8" – 1" inches. On average I have mostly seen legs that are ¼" shorter. The leg gets jammed upwards into the hip socket. The body shifts over the leg which then crunches the low back, hip, and leg together. Over time this area will become hard because it is being crunched into itself. Now it is an easy area to pull and one may have chronic low back pain until they learn to stretch and flex their leg out of their hip socket.

When you walk on one leg the foot must point outwards more to support all the weight. This makes the outside of the leg tighter which will pull the hips backward and shift the pelvis to the injured leg side. This will affect the foundation of the spine and it will start to curve, possibly causing scoliosis. The spine will continue to curve all the way up the spine and then curve the other way possibly causing cervical neck pain. So, if you have a chronic neck pain on the right side of the neck then you may not be flexing your left toe (which would d be the short leg). When one leg is shorter than the other it is best just to concentrate on this shorter leg. Step Point 4 is best used to lengthen a short leg. This requires hitting the big toe and lengthening your leg behind you. If you work on these issues without flexing the toe, your symptoms of low back pain, hip pain and scoliosis will continually need to be treated.[1]

If your injury has never been massaged you may find that the area may still have some hardness around it, and this is scar tissue. Massage techniques such as cross fiber friction, which is rubbing the opposite length of the muscle fibers, will help break up scar tissue bringing in circulation and cellular regeneration.[2] Also flexing these scar tissue areas will help break them up.

Another technique that I use is a roller or yoga ball. I sit on the ball and roll it around till I feel a painful stiffness. The muscle is stiff because the muscle is stuck. So, I will roll it around and then flex my hip into the ball. Pain is due to the muscle being out of place. When you flex the muscle into place it will reset to its original position and then it finally gets to rest.

Fan Belt of Cause and Effect

When our foot transitions from Step Points 1-2 to Step Points 3-4, we are pushing on the outside of the foot transitioning to the inside foot. The fan belt analogy is showing that if one side is being tightened the other side is being pulled. Usually the side that is being pulled is where the pain is. Any appendage has a set of muscles that pull the

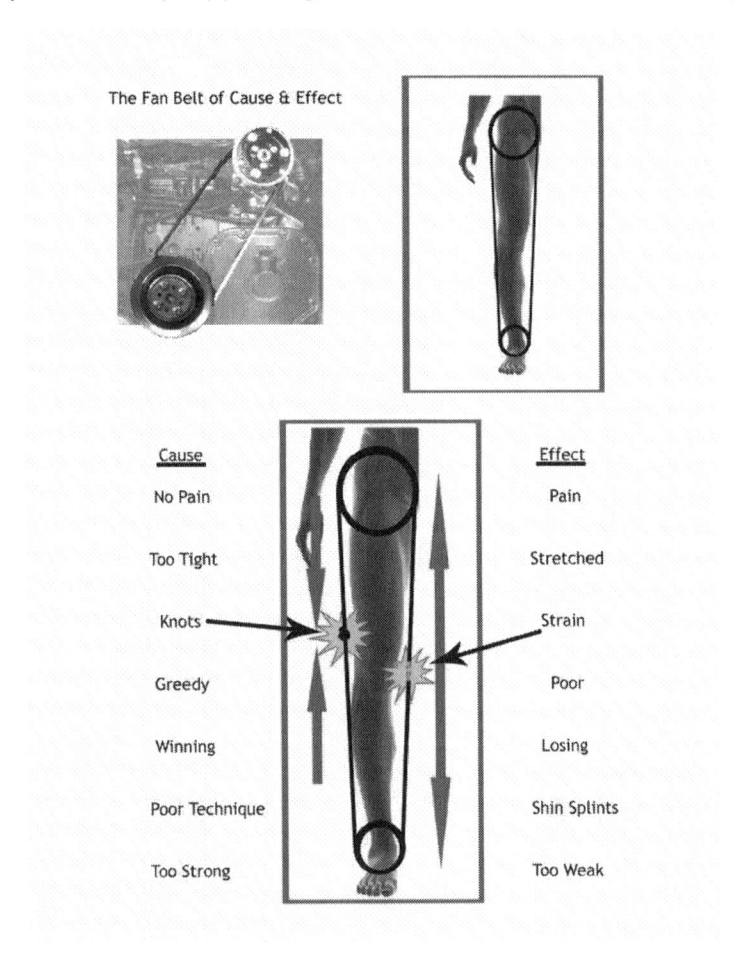

The Fan Belt of Cause & Effect

Cause	Effect
No Pain	Pain
Too Tight	Stretched
Knots	Strain
Greedy	Poor
Winning	Losing
Poor Technique	Shin Splints
Too Strong	Too Weak

appendage one way and then another set of muscles pull the appendage the opposite direction.

If we are walking on the outside of your feet only then you are tightening your IT Band (outside leg muscles) and straining/pulling your inside leg muscles. If you are standing on the back of your heels then you are straining the front of your legs. Both scenarios will lead to tight hips and symptoms like sciatica and low back pain occur.[3]

To bring the fan belt of balance back inline one must flex the strained muscles. So, if you are used to walking on the outside of feet then you really need to focus on flexing your inside leg muscles when your leg is behind you.

Chapter Eight

The Core

Engaging your Internal Muscles improves Posture

I have found that yoga instructors are very adamant about engaging your core. The core is your lower abdomen and hips. There is a lot of action that takes place here and being strong in your core is very important. In most yoga poses being strong in your core helps with being able to hold some of the poses. The core helps you twist, stand

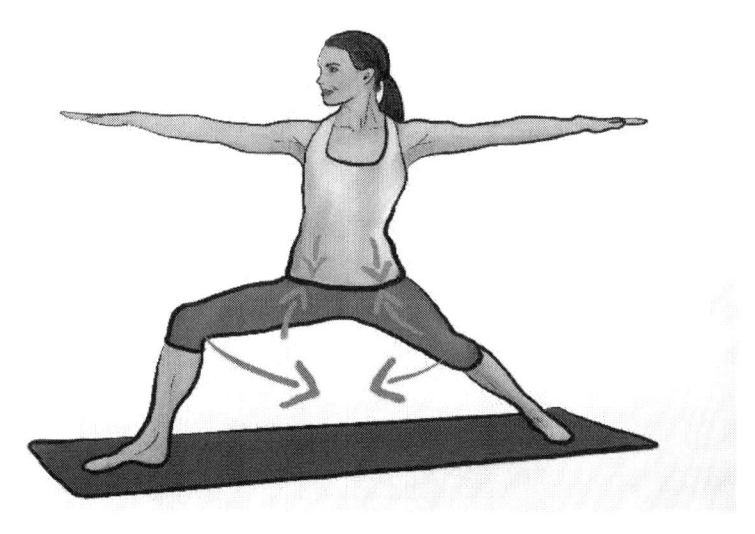

Warrior Pose

up, and lift your legs. And of course, it is crucial to engage your core while walking.[1]

Most yoga instructors will want you to engage your core while doing certain poses like chair and warrior pose. But the next step is focusing on your core with your inner legs at the same time. When walking, this action of engaging your core happens when your legs are apart like taking a walking stride or when doing the yoga warrior pose.

Most of the time bad posture starts with our bodies getting tired and we slump down into ourselves and slouch. Sometimes while driving in the morning I move my rearview mirror up and then by the evening I must move it down because I have "shrunk" throughout the day.

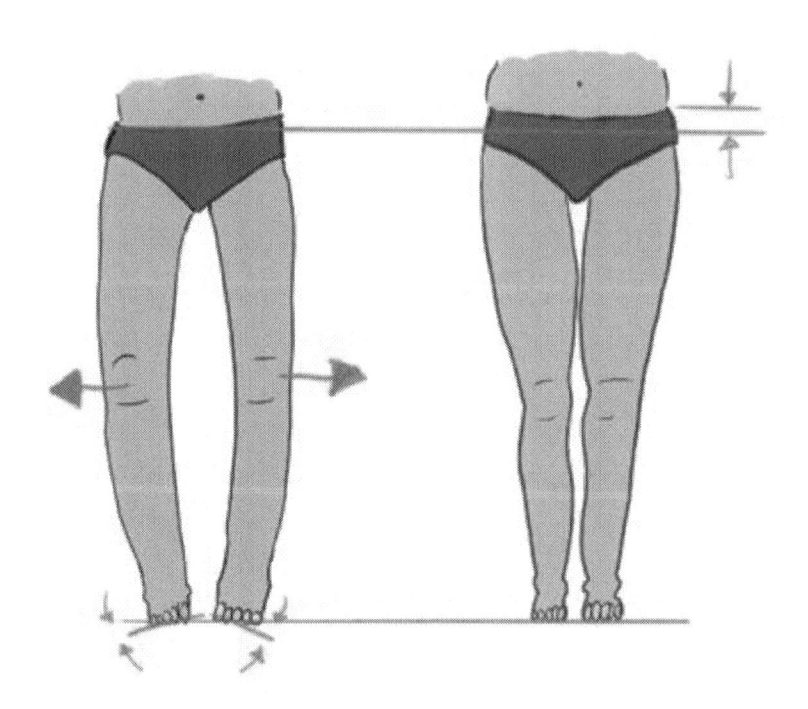

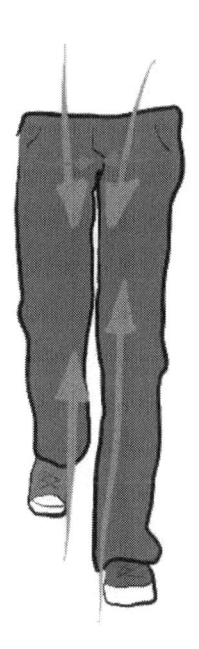

By engaging your core, you are helping to strengthen the inner muscle groups that hold you upright. I have noticed that there is a space between your hips and lower abdomen. I have noticed that my torso will slump into my hips. This in turn will bow my hip sockets out and my legs turn out and then I am walking on the outer edges of my feet. If I am strong in my core while engaging my inner legs, my torso lifts and my feet become flat to the ground. I also notice my ankles have less pressure on them and if feels like I just lost 20 lbs. When we are off balance and have bad posture, our ankles and feet must make up for the imbalance. So, when you improve your posture, you will feel less pressure on your feet and ankles. Those that have ankle pain will want to pay special attention to this detail as it is likely your sinking posture is creating your pain.[2]

When we are in a bad posture and not engaging our core, we are not standing on our bones. Instead we are "standing" on our muscles to make up the difference. Muscles do not like doing the job of bones. If the muscles do the skeletal work due to bad posture, they become very hard. I call this "bone tight" because your muscles become so tight they feel as hard as a bone.

Accessing your core does take some practice. It is a difficult concept to get at first. In yoga class, I heard the instructor talk about the core for years and for the longest time I had no idea what they were talking about. Flexing your core is difficult to see. It is an internal flex, the center of your gravity. In some martial arts they aim for your core. This is the area just below your belly button. We would play a game called "push hands". This game is played by standing flat footed and you try and push each other over. If you can push the "magic button" (the core, below the belly button) you will easily push the other person over. The core is the internal stabilizer of balance.

When you are about to access Step Point 3 (when stepping from Step Point 2 to 3), this is the point at which to engage the core of your inner hips and abdomen. When your leg is moving behind you, that is when you are flexing your inner leg and your core at the same time. Utilizing this technique will help push your shoulders and your head back into the right alignment, which will give you a stronger upright posture.

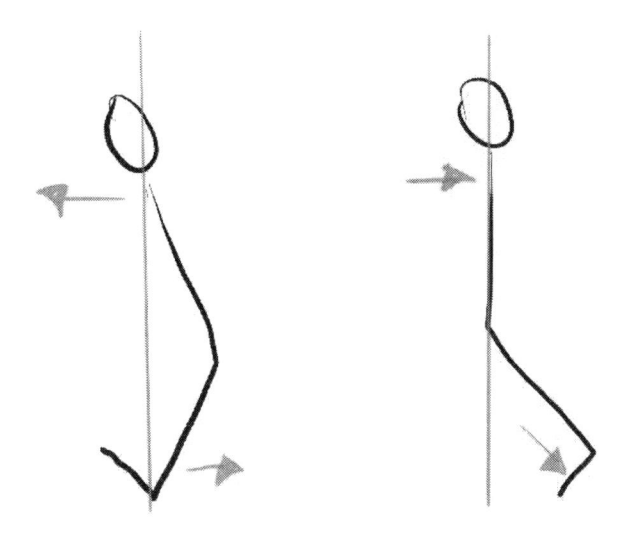

Pregnancy & Holding a Baby

Children do bring joy to the world; however, it does not bring joy to your body. Your body does take a toll for creating life. In the "Toes Pointed Forward" Chapter, we go into the detail of having your feet pointed forward to prevent low back pain. Unfortunately, this cannot be avoided when growing a fetus. Inevitably as the fetus grows your center of weight changes and you are going to have to point your feet outwards to counter the expanding weight for your own balance. Ideally before a lady gets pregnant it would be best to develop and master the hip muscles and get them in shape to carry the new imbalance. However, this is not always predictable.

The link below has some good yoga exercise by searching for "Prenatal hip Exercises in Yoga".

https://www.healthline.com/health/pregnancy/stretches#14

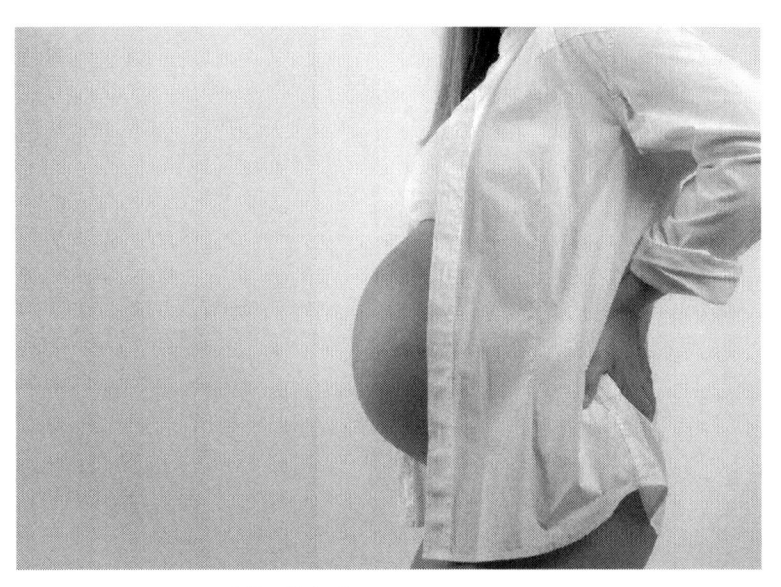

https://pixabay.com

In each of these exercises they are encouraging opening and strengthening the hip muscles. This is great, however, the important muscles to focus on are the inside leg muscles. Specific muscles like the psoas and iliacus assist with lifting the thigh forward.[3]

So, these muscles will be overstretched as the baby grows. These muscles can also be strained because they are doing a lot of support to hold the developing baby. If you do not engage them to keep them strong and pliable, then they will harden. There will be a tendency for ladies to lean backwards to counter the growing baby. This however will tighten the hamstrings and further stress the back of the hips likely enhancing sciatica and low back pain. When you engage the front of the hips you will help to relieve some of the tension from the tailbone area.

In each of the yoga hip exercises it is important to flex and tone the inside leg muscles. When doing a lunge or a squat engaging the inside leg muscles is imperative to stabilizing your hips. This will also pull your center of weight forward instead of falling backwards.[4]

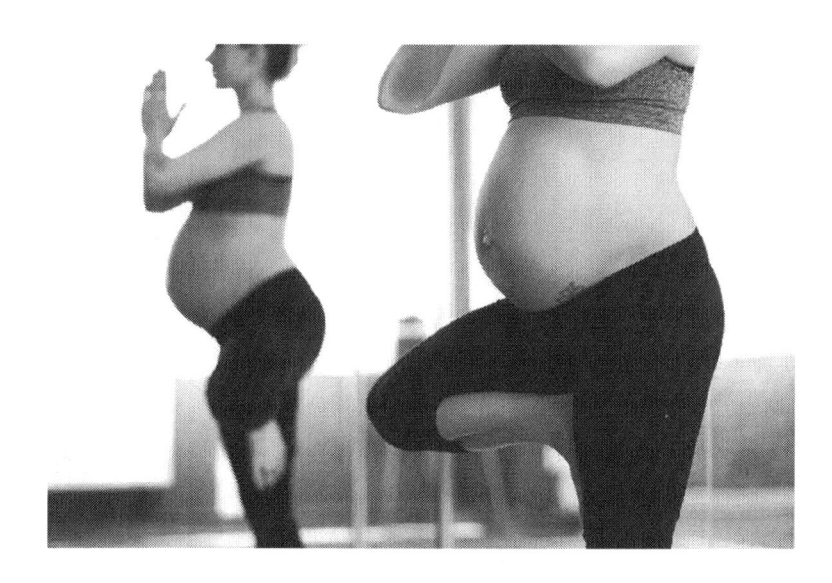

Photo by freestocks.org from Pexels

While pregnant the relaxin hormone is increased making your joints and ligaments more mobile. So, if things are moving around it is important to keep things toned so joints don't move too far out of place or get extremely overstretched. After child birth hip muscles may be in some cases way out of position. Now the yoga hip exercises are more important to realign your hips while the relaxin hormone is digressing.[5]

Holding a baby has its own issues. Often, we will put the baby on one hip to carry them around while we can use the other arm to do tasks. When it comes to balance it is important to switch arms. When we use the same arm and hip to carry the baby that hip will jet outwards, up, and forward. This can lead to your hips to be at an angle. The pelvis can twist thus increasing or not resolving the on-going sacrum-low back pain. Often the inner legs and abdomen area is not in shape, so these issues can further exacerbate the pain.[6]

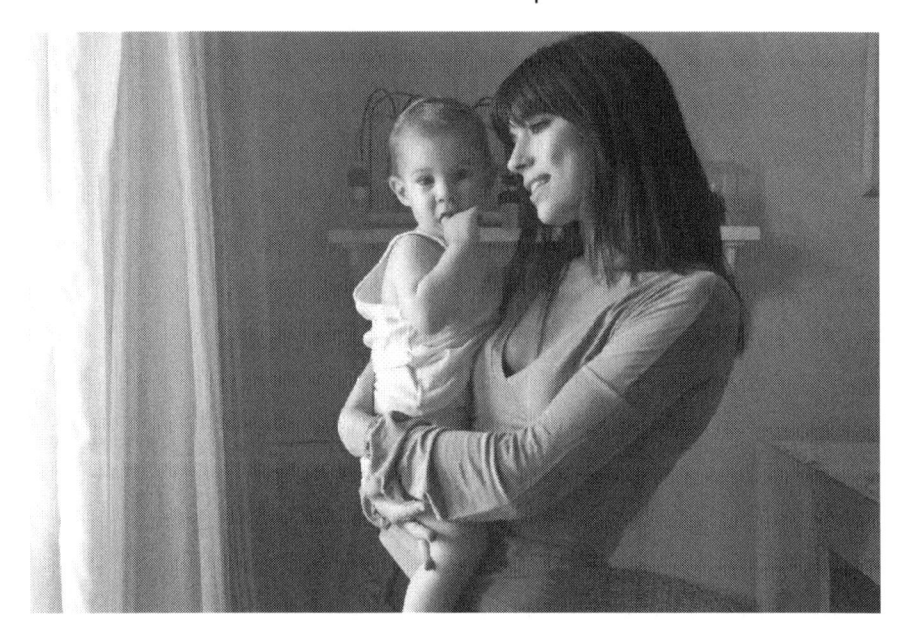

Photo by Bruce mars from Pexels

So, while the baby is growing up you will have lots of time to walk them in a stroller. This is a good time to engage the inner legs and strengthen your hip muscles. Flex your abdomen and really push off that inner foot to open and tone your inner hips.

I recommend getting one of those jogger strollers while taking walks. With a typical stroller, it is difficult to take a long walking stride because the handle is often too close to you and you will kick the stroller. So, things I did was walk beside the stroller, so I could extend my legs.

Chapter Nine

Posture
Putting it all together

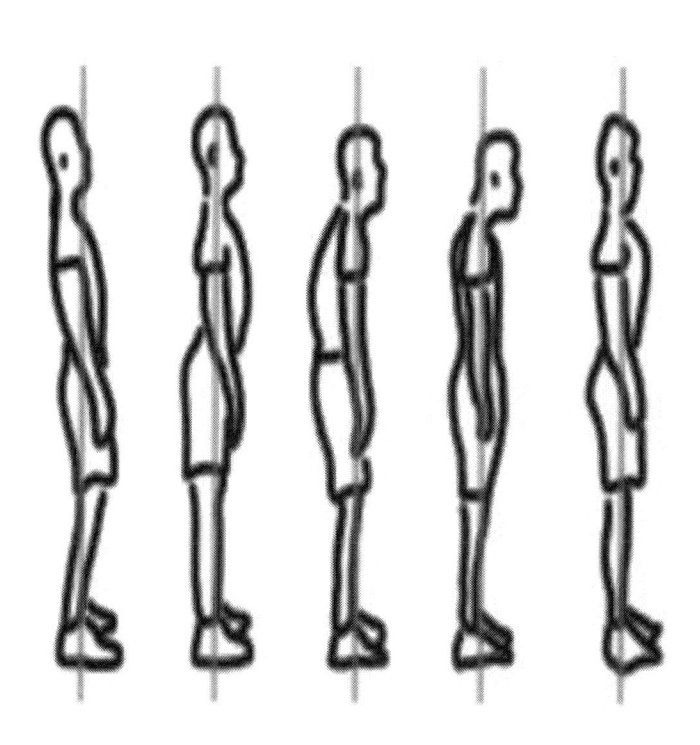

There are many ways to have a posture that creates pain. They depend on past injuries, your mental outlook, repetitive activities, inner strength, and body awareness.

This second picture is a very common posture that I see. The toes are pointed outward and most of the weight is on the back of the legs. This will lead to tight hamstrings and a stiff neck.

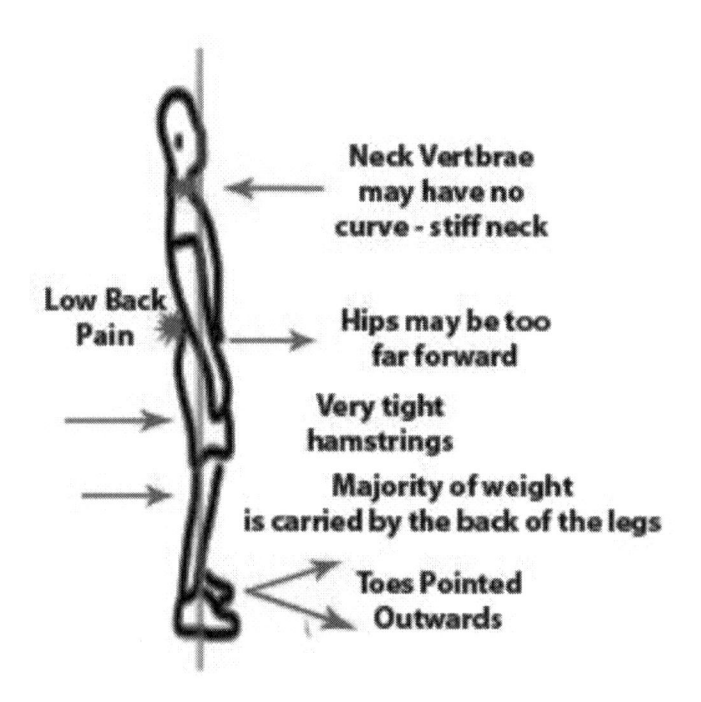

Neck Vertbrae may have no curve - stiff neck

Low Back Pain

Hips may be too far forward

Very tight hamstrings

Majority of weight is carried by the back of the legs

Toes Pointed Outwards

The next posture is opposite of the last where instead of leaning on the back of their legs they are leaning on the front of the legs. This will arch the back backwards. Their neck may have no curve, which may create a very tight neck.

Lordosis refers to your natural lordotic curve, which is the curve in your lower back. But if your curve arches too far inward, it can create lower back pain. This can lead to an increase of pressure on the spine, because the alignment of the discs are off-center.[1]

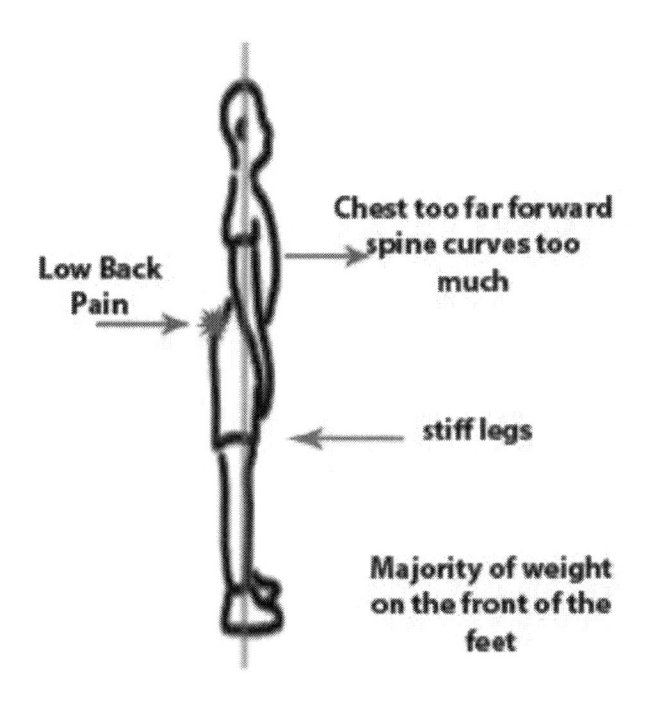

Low Back Pain

Chest too far forward
spine curves too much

stiff legs

Majority of weight on the front of the feet

Next is a posture that happens to a lot of computer people. Often at a desk, people will have this position while sitting. Then they stand up and walk around still in the same posture. When we are driving a car we are also in this same posture. It's important to engage your feet and let them push your shoulders back. When one does not use their feet their back will round forward and the head will jet forward. Now the front of the neck is holding up the head. So this person will have a very tight front of the neck and the back of the neck will be over stretched. This is one of the variables of headaches.

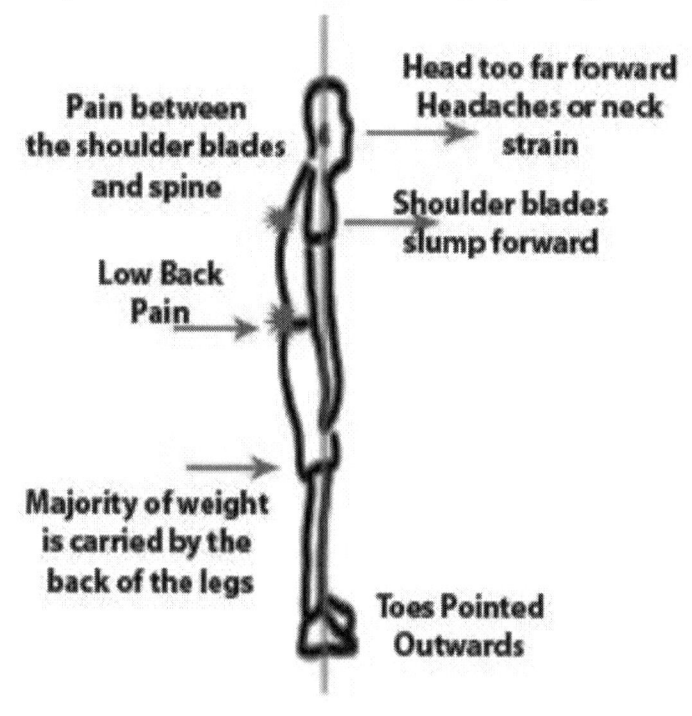

The most common form of kyphosis is from poor posture. Kyphosis is when the spine is curved forward. Patients with postural kyphosis can conscientiously correct the curve by standing up straight. For these patients there is no actual structural abnormality of the spine and their curve is unlikely to progress.[2]

Next, those that walk on the front of their feet or have their toes pointed inwards will have this posture. Their hips will be the first thing that enters the room. The hips and legs fall forward while the torso and head try and keep up.

Overpronation and toes pointed inwards will make the core of the body weak. This will make the hips slump forward, the torso will fall backwards, and then the head will jet forward.

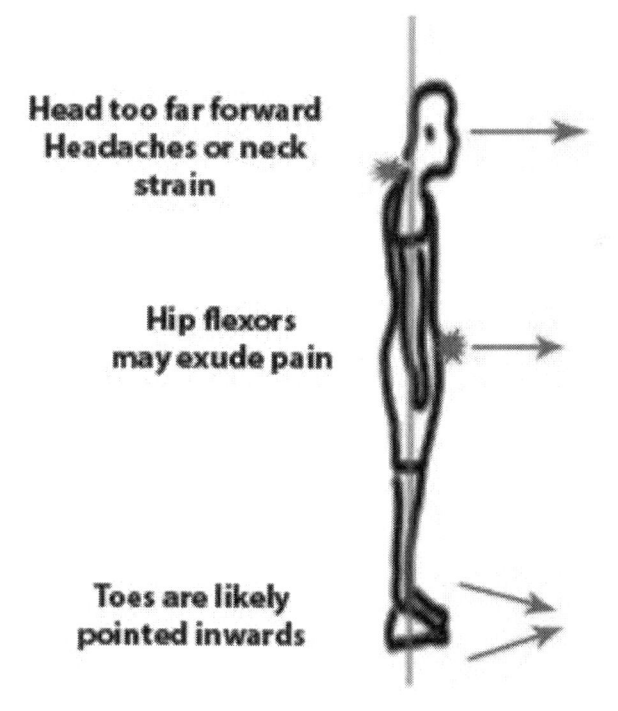

**Head too far forward
Headaches or neck strain**

**Hip flexors
may exude pain**

**Toes are likely
pointed inwards**

This is a demonstration that there is no absolute way to have bad posture. There are many ways a body can contort. To stop painful bad posture, one must have awareness of yourself and noticing when your body pain occurs. Often the peak of bad posture happens at about ¾ of the way through the day. This is when you are a little exhausted and not paying attention to your posture technique. When you are using muscles that do not help you with posture these muscles will fatigue faster. Therefore, people squirm and wind up in strange positions like sitting on one leg or using one arm to hold up their head. When you start to strengthen your posture and sit and stand with better authority to correct your posture, the muscles that you have been not using will fatigue faster. So, it is important to know which way you are standing so when the bad posture pain creeps in you know which way to flex your body and change this bad posture habit into a good helpful healing posture. Over time when you are aware of when you are falling into a bad posture you will have the awareness to flex into a better position that supports your weak and underdeveloped posture muscles.

Chapter Ten

Not all Pain is created equal - The Case for how Osteoarthritis is Created

Osteoarthritis is the most common type of arthritis. When the cartilage – the slick, cushioning surface on the ends of bones – wears away, bone rubs against bone, causing pain, swelling and stiffness. Over time, joints can lose strength and pain may become chronic. Risk factors include excess weight, family history, age and previous injury (an anterior cruciate ligament, or ACL, tear, for example).[1]

~ArthritisFoundation.org

Often the suggested treatments I see out there are is, stop doing it, lose weight, don't go up or down hills, avoid injuries, and repetitive movements.

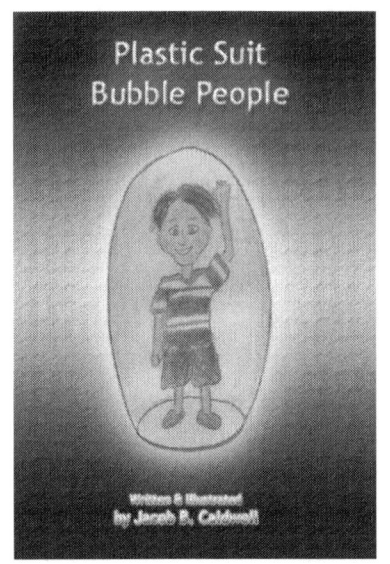

So just live in a bubble, don't do anything and everything will be fine. I wrote a children's book called the "Plastic Suit Bubble People" for those people. Of course, it does not end well for the bubble people.[2]

I believe there are solutions everywhere and we need more of the "do this stuff" to repair ourselves rather than just "stop everything". So, let's look at how some of these issues are created and the solutions that are given to retain optimum health. If we do not understand how an issue is created, then we are just guessing to what the solutions are and when we are in pain we have no time for guessing.

Arthritis is often defined as a compressed joint, or inflammatory response that exudes heat and swelling. These are symptoms and we must look at why are they happening. Inflammation mean "in flames", something is irritated so let's figure out why it is irritated? Often the therapy is just using an anti-inflammation drug to put out the fire. This does work, but in my opinion, it should be used as an emergency tool on occasion, not like a daily vitamin.

Lack of Range of Motion (ROM) – Repetitive Motion

One of the ways a joint can be inflamed is due to lack of range of motion. Very few of us have jobs where we can use all the various motions that are appendages express. Often in our jobs we are constantly doing repetitive motion type jobs. Cashiers in grocery stores can get carpal tunnel due to pulling produce from the conveyor belt and twist their arm through the scanner. Computer workers are pushing a computer mouse button or keyboard all day while sitting. As a massage therapist we are bending over people and applying the same squeezing motion while massaging people.

These repetitive motion activities add up over time. To relive stiffness in a joint it is best to exercise a joint in both directions. However, when we are doing a repetitive motion we are only flexing our appendages in one direction for a long period of time without going the other direction. When we are only going in one direction for a long period of time that muscle group starts to become strong and dominant and stuck in the direction it is constantly being used in. The muscle group that pulls the joint the opposing direction starts to become flaccid and underdeveloped and will be pulled and overstretched by the constant overused muscle group. It becomes a tug-o-war within the joint itself. When one muscle group is stronger than its opposing muscle group the appendage will start to favor the stronger muscle group and the joint will start to be "bent" out of place. When a joint is not in the correct alignment it will be stretched in an awkward way and start to become irritated. The joint will begin to "harden" to protect itself from the misalignment of the stress on the joint. When a body part is stressed it will harden and become tight, so it won't break. Now when these muscle and joints have hardened they need to be properly "warmed up" with stretches or slow impact movements. If these stretches are not done and we go right into the repetitive motion again you will compound the microtearing which may create more hardening of the joint, muscles, and soft tissue. When a muscle is constantly used in a repetitive motion it will start to acquire microtears. When a muscle is worked and strained it breaks down which is microtearing.[23] This is normal to strength building. Rest and therapy will assist in the rebuilding of the muscle, but the problem occurs when we do not rest the muscle enough so that it is repaired. When the muscle is not repaired enough It will start to develop a small scar tissue effect. This scar tissue is a quick band-aide to repair the muscle. Scar tissue is very fibrous and strong; however, it also will restrict movement and keep the injured area tight.

So, creating a joint that is stuck in one position most of the time is one of the variables for osteoarthritis, which is part of the definition that contributes to a compressed joint.

Dehydration

Check out the "What is Water Chapter" because water is not created equal. A big part of societies issues can be linked to dehydration. Water moves through our bodies through the lymph system. Water really needs to be seen as a transportation vehicle for delivering minerals to cells and eliminating cellular waste. Our muscles are like a wad of rubber bands. If you apply some soapy water to a string of rubber bands they will slide effortlessly. But when you take away the water the rubber bands are forced to rub against each other, they will start to heat up and then stick to each other. This is what happens when you are dehydrated. The muscles will stick to each other and if you are in a repetitive motion job all day while dehydrated, those muscles will stick in that position. Which means your joints will be stuck out of position as well.

If you are dehydrated all week and you have only been doing your repetitive motion at work, when it comes time for the weekend to be the "Weekend Warrior" or wrestle with the kids, you may be on the verge of creating an injury. In athletics your body may go in different directions than it has been in all week. So, if your muscles have hardened into your computer mouse arm position, while being dehydrated, it will become very easy to injure yourself. Pulled muscles will be common and chronic issues will persist because you are not pliable enough to bend in multiple actions because you are frozen in place due to repetitive motion while being dehydrated.

If you injure yourself while being dehydrated your muscles will stick together from the impact. Your body will stay in this stuck position. If you are hydrated while being injured, you have a better chance of your muscles retracting to their original positions. A deep tissue massage does unravel many of these stuck out-of-place muscles, however muscles will undo way easier when you are hydrated.

Dehydration is another one of the variables that is attributed to osteoarthritis. When there is lack of lubrication and circulation this can lead to the deterioration of a joint.

Synovial Fluid

Synovial fluid contributes significant stabilizing effects as an adhesive seal that freely permits sliding motion between cartilaginous surfaces while effectively resisting distracting forces.[3]

-Frederick A. Matsen III, M.D.

Synovial fluid is the lubricant of the joint. When a joint is under pressure and then released it acts like a hydraulic pump. The pressure pushes the synovial fluid into the cartilage and delivers nutrients into the cartilage. Just like a hydraulic pump to deliver the nutrients into the cartilage the full motion of the joint needs to often reach a full extension so it can deliver a force to push the nutrients into the cartilage.[4]

However, if a joint is not exercised often or with enough constant force the nutrients will not be delivered. Also, the motion of the appendage helps pump new synovial fluid with new nutrients into the joint. The more a joint is used the rate of production of more synovial fluid will be available.[5] If a muscle group is compressed due to dehydration or stuck in a position of repetitive motion the cartilage may not receive enough nutrients and may start to deteriorate. This is one of the beginning variables to create osteoarthritis.[6]

This information leads to the importance of exercising. Joint movement under some light to heavy resistance is necessary for joint and cartilage health. When we wake in the morning our bodies are a little stiff and the more we move they loosen up because the synovial fluid level is increased. It is recommended that if one is about to do some more excessive recreational exercising like snowboarding, rock climbing, or flag football that one has a stretching routine or light workout to get your body ready to move in any direction. As we age it is more and more important to make the body pliable so that we can prevent injuries and get our body ready so that fun activities can remain to be fun.

Nutrition - genetics

If there is not enough nutrition that one is consuming, then it doesn't matter what the flexibility or constriction that the joint may be under. According to Dr. Joel Wallach, ND raging osteoporosis is due to a lack of nutrients to rebuild the bone and cartilage structure. Vitamin D helps absorb calcium into the body. However, this calcium may not be absorbed due to excessive inflammation from being gluten intolerant. "Only four stomach animals have the biology to eat grains only", says Dr. Wallach who is a Naturopathic Doctor (ND) and has a Doctorate in Veterinary Medicine (DVM). This will inflame the intestines and your body will have trouble absorbing nutrition let alone calcium. Lack of absorbing calcium creates kidney stones, bone spurs, calcium deposits especially where tendons and ligaments attach. So, improper nutrition along with inflammatory foods will lead to your bone and cartilage not to be replenished or replaced.[7]

Everyone that dies of natural causes, dies of a Mineral Deficiency.

- Dr. Joel Wallach, ND

You are not what you eat, but what you absorb.

- Dr. Joel Wallach, ND

According to Dr. Jerry Tennant, MD in his book "Healing is Voltage", he talks about that the body needs to achieve a certain amount of voltage to repair itself. He points to minerals to help in aiding the increase in voltage. Minerals are a metal that conducts energy much like fiber optics. Water is the transportation device to deliver minerals. Unfortunately tap water contains very little minerals and has too many chemicals in it to be considered useful as a source of hydration and contain the appropriate level of mineral content. Usually minerals need to be added and chemicals need to be filtered for water to be useful to any living being.

So, if a body is not receiving enough minerals to have the appropriate voltage to repair itself this could lead to a system wide degeneration. The necessary repairs needed to maintain the body will slowly fall behind. This can lead to degeneration of bones, the wearing down of cartilage, and muscles and tendons not getting proper maintenance.

If you have a body with a continuous acidic or low pH your body will pull minerals out of your bones. This is another variable to the creation of osteoarthritis.

"You probably wouldn't notice being in a slightly acidic state — it isn't associated with obvious immediate symptoms. But if it goes on for a long time, it can slowly lead to osteoporosis and other degenerative health disorders because bone-protecting minerals have been used up to restore pH balance.[8]

-- Dr. Susan E. Brown

(The "What is Water" Chapter will go into the importance of pH.)

Mental Stress

When your body is under stress it acts like a hardener. Whatever position you are in under stress for an amount of time your body will harden in that position.

In my massage sessions I use a lot of Range of Motion and Passive Stretching Techniques. This helps me to see where the body is tight and then this can bring awareness to the client so then they can relax their body.

Often where things are tight is the same position that one is in the most stress at the time. It's when people do a different activity like helping someone move, go rock climbing, ride a bike, or step off a curb wrong is when they injure themselves. Because of the stressful position their body has been in, the muscle loses its pliability to suddenly move in different directions. Often people will blame the activity of that moment which irritated the new inflammatory injury. But really it is because the body is under mental stress for a long period of time is the true culprit.[9]

The human body is designed to heal itself. This cannot occur unless it is in a state of homeostasis, so the body will do what is necessary to try to maintain this balance. Homeostasis is the state of balance when all the supporting internal fluids are at their ideal healthy level.[24] When the body is in stress or injured the body will go out of the homeostatic balance. It will use minerals like calcium, potassium and sodium, which are alkalizing minerals to keep this balance. Therefore, a person may end up with problems due to the decrease of these minerals, such as osteoporosis from the leeching of calcium.[25]

When we are in stress we shrink into ourselves. We are micro-flexing and holding our body still with shallow breathing.[10] Fluids are not able to hydrate, and the extra adrenaline produces an acidic environment. When your body is in a consistent acidic environment it deteriorates the body. The healing response will not kick in because when we are in a stress state our bodies are in a fear state. This means our bodies will not repair if we are in more of a fear state than a resting state. The stress and fear state are useful when running from a tiger. However, after we have run from the tiger we need our bodies to repair so we can be ready to run again if we need to. However, if one is in a constant state of stress, with not enough rest to repair one's self, the body may fall apart.

It is important to have outlets to destress. Take time for recreation, viewing art, take in a show, or get a massage. Getting your mind off things helps your mind rest so you can have a fresh new look on things later. Getting stressed out takes a toll on your body. Resting is doing. Take a break. Even God rested on the 7th day, you should too.

Scar Tissue and Taking care of Old Injuries

Scar tissue is a fibrous tissue that works very fast to quickly heal an injury. Unfortunately, because it is so tough it will harden the muscle in about the same position that it was injured.[11]

So, if you did not take care of your injury after the pain went away it is possible the muscle is still stuck in the same injured position. This can act and feel the same way a dehydrated repetitive motion muscle is stuck. The appendage and muscle group may have limited motion within the joint because of the stiffness and may lead to a different injury or easily lead to reinjuring the same muscle group. So, a stiff joint with too much scar tissue can lead to osteoarthritis because the joint is not being moved to its full capacity and it is limited. Over time, the joint will not be nourished, and the muscles will not reclaim its elasticity.

Minor injuries can have their own lingering consequences. They may not be serious enough to get a cast, splint, or qualify for a rehabilitation therapy series. They can be easily be ignored and we just limb around and tolerate it. If you have had something like a severely sprained ankle or knee injury over time these issues can be a time bomb waiting. One can wait for decades before an old injury becomes an issue. A joint that has been compromised will become tight and harden. Some of these knee and hip replacement issues could be the result of not properly rehabbing the injury. It will be tight for such a long time and the supporting soft tissue has been holding the joint still. This compresses the joint and the cushion is gone thus creating the "bone on bone" phenomenon.[26]

Rest to Repair

Ultimately, we want equal flexion and extension with each of our joints and use the appropriate muscles to be exercised in the right direction. Over a period of misuse, this is how a lot of these inflammatory issues occur. Our bodies have a high tolerance of letting you go out of balance for a certain period. Often in sports, in an event, sometimes our bodies are contorting in all sorts of ways. We can get away with a strange move or two, however, if there is a movement that is too extreme or is constantly compromising the joint without a proper rest, it will lead to an inflammatory or chronic nerve pain.[19]

When we are overworking a muscle that is creating inflammation our body is in the flight response. Which means there is an emergency and the body will be in stress. When we align our joint and flex them in the proper position homeostasis we will begin to heal. However, if a joint is constantly under stress and out of position it will not be in a space of healing.[20]

"The solution to overactivation of our fight or flight response is simple: when we take the time to exercise our relaxation response "muscle" we will enjoy the beneficial physiological, biochemical and mental effects. These beneficial effects are measurable whether we believe in the relaxation response or not".[21]

-Neil F. Neimark, M.D

Arthritis is caused by the body's reaction to an increase in joint pressure. This can be caused by several factors including: immobility, lack of exercise, or a misaligned joint especially in the spine. This causes stress of the joints and forces them to support a greater responsibility than they are designed to. The symptoms caused by arthritis are your body's way of telling you that something in the body is not right.[22]

Homeostasis is about balance. When we enter homoeostasis, the body will start to heal. When we are out of homeostasis and under stress we go into a flight response and the body is in an emergency state which is what inflammation is signaling. Proper rest and joint alignment will achieve homeostasis. Joint pain and inflammation are a signal your muscle technique is not in the correct position compromising your joints.

Breaking up Scar Tissue to Promote Muscle Growth

After an injury if we would like to progress being healed, we need to repair the muscle. This takes place after the inflammation has gone away and the muscle has repaired. After the inflammation has gone down, we may have no pain response from the injury, however, the injured muscle is still stiff which may be scar tissue. We need to crunch through the scar tissue and flex our muscles. Often with an injury people will just not use the muscles and will compensate by using other surrounding muscles.

Flexing our muscles helps bring back elasticity and encourages the muscle to rebuild itself. In the StretchFlex Chapter in the back of the book talks about this technique. When we stretch an injured muscle we also need to flex it in the other direction. This will help reestablish the muscles position. Pain is because the muscles are out of place and so we need to flex them back into place. I have found it difficult to just stretch a muscle back into position by itself. So, when you stretch and feel the pain, then you want to find that pain and flex the pain away. When you do this, I have found that half of the pain goes away and stretching is not so torturous.[12]

So, if we do not flex our muscles into the correct position and reestablish our full range of motion, break up the scar tissue, over time this is another cause of osteoarthritis.[13,14,15,16,17]

Excess Weight

Continual excess weight can act on a joint just like a dehydrated-repetitive-motioned-scar-tissued appendage. Due to the extra weight, joints are constantly compressed, and the surrounding soft tissue will harden. This will cause constant wear and tear without the proper rest which minimizes elasticity of weight bearing joints.

Walking off-center and misalignment will have the same effect on your body as excessive weight. Our bones are meant for structural support and our muscles are for turning and moving our body. When we are not walking upright on our bones, then we are using our muscles as the structural support. Soon these muscles will turn in to what I call "bone tight". They are so tight that the muscles will feel as hard as bones.

It takes 6.25 lbs./sq. of pressure to distort tissue.[18] So, when we are adding more weight to ourselves we are increasing the pressure on our soft tissues and joints. So, excessive weight is another one of the variables that can contribute to osteoarthritis.

What is Stiffness?

If you have been doing a repetitive action or non-action like standing or sitting for a while. When you begin to first move you may be stuck/stiff at first. The level of stiffness intensity will be how long have you been in that position. Also, the level at which how well you are hydrated will be a factor.

As mentioned before, repetitive motion, the motion of flexing in a direction without flexing the opposite direction, will add to the intensity or your stiffness. Add dehydration to the equation and you will be even more stiff. Time and dehydration without stretching or drinking enough water will compound your stiff joints. Being dehydrated may also affect the levels of your synovial fluid in your joints. Synovial fluid helps lubricate joints and if there is not enough water in your system this can also cause stiffness.[28]

The Pain Scale - TIME

There are many variables that come together to create chronic issues. One of them is Time. Your body has a lot of tolerance to absorb and allow you to be out of balance for a certain amount of time. However, repetitive movement over a certain amount of time will compound your issues.

Some of the chronic issues we have are from tasks that you do all the time. Recently, I had a computer worker with a "mysterious" shoulder issue. She has been a computer worker for over a decade, so she has accumulated some tight shoulders. One day she was walking her dog and the dog lunged and he yanked her shoulder. The one act of the dog lunging could be pointed to as the initial problem. But what was the real problem was the decade of repetitive motion of the keyboard that really set up the chronic issue. Like a frog being slowly boiled in a pot the frog does not feel anything. Just like a computer user who sits in the same position does not feel the compounding tightness from the repetitive motion. Over time the computer user will become tight in this position and the tolerance to bend a different and sudden action will "break" the tight muscles. This will cause a lot of inflammation and stress on the soft tissues like nerves, ligaments and tendons.

The Pain Scale

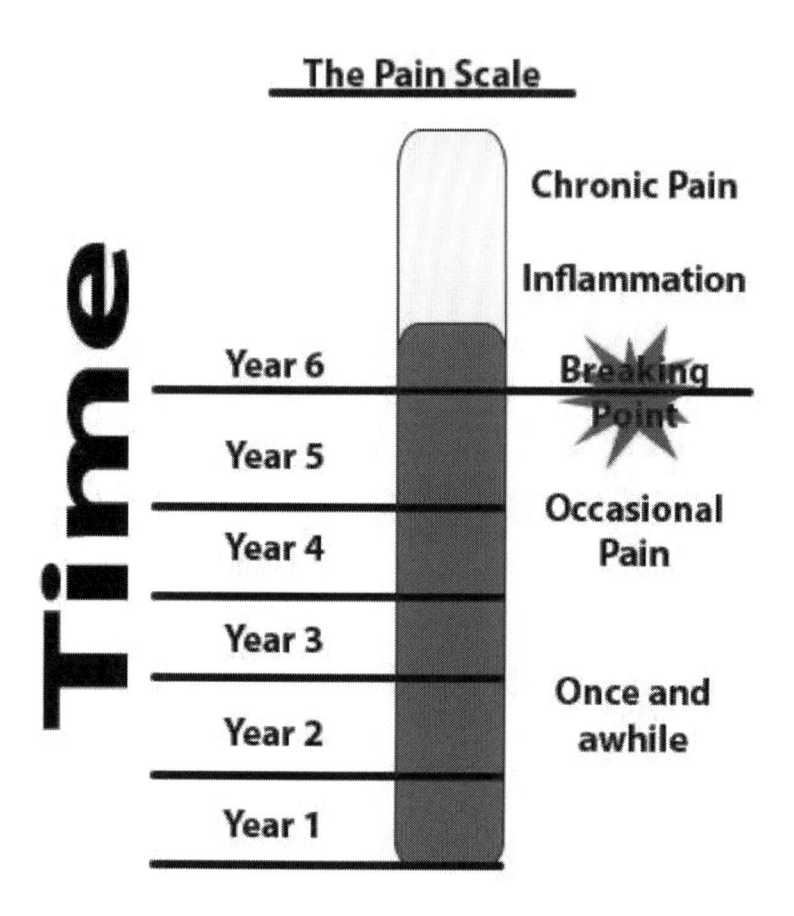

```
Time

Year 6 ─────── Chronic Pain
              Inflammation
Year 5 ─────── Breaking Point

Year 4 ─────── Occasional Pain

Year 3 ───────

Year 2 ─────── Once and awhile

Year 1 ───────
```

The Pain Scale - Accumulating Variables add up

To create a chronic condition requires a lot of variables to add up. Since the body allows us to bend the rules for a bit, the body does have a breaking point. The body allows you to stay ahead of the pain if you hydrate, meditate, counter stretch, and consume good nutrition. However, if you do not do any of the balancing therapies to counter repetitive stress this will add up over time.

There are stories of grandfather and grandma smokers who smoked for 70 years and lived to be 90+. However, we find out that these people worked outside, ate homegrown food, and were around few chemicals. So, this natural way of living countered some of the bad smoking habits and they were able to live longer than most who may have grown up in the city working at a chemical company, eating fast food for lunch every day, and sitting in front of the TV for hours.

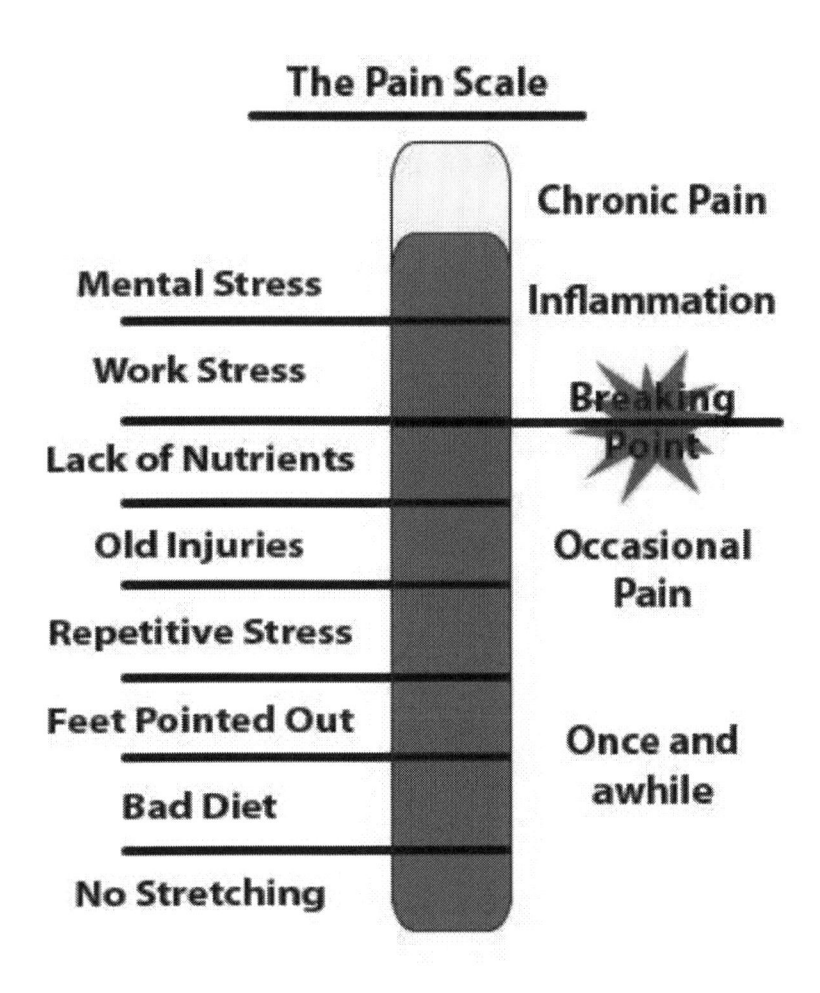

The Pain Scale

- Mental Stress
- Work Stress
- Lack of Nutrients
- Old Injuries
- Repetitive Stress
- Feet Pointed Out
- Bad Diet
- No Stretching

Chronic Pain

Inflammation

Breaking Point

Occasional Pain

Once and awhile

So, there is really no way to say an issue will happen to one person will happen to everyone else. There is a sum of variables that need to happen. Most diseases and chronic pain issues will have a variety of issues that will add up. Specifically, low back pain has many ways of appearing. One office worker after a decade of sitting may have low back symptoms. Where another computer worker gets the same intense low back issue after 2 years. Same job, same ergonomic set up, same level of pain intensity. The difference could be the first computer worker took better care of themselves and likely had fewer accumulating variables. Perhaps they ate better food, better frequency of drinking water, or the 2nd worker had their toes pointed more outward than the first worker.

One person can have chronic back pain due to posture, stress, and a bad diet. Another person can have the same level of back pain due to repetitive stress and then stepped off a curb wrong. The goal is to lessen the severity of each of the variables that add to the climbing pain scale. Simple solutions are that computer workers are starting to stand up half the day rather than sit 100% of the day. People are taking more breaks and walking around. Ingesting more water and consuming less dehydration liquid like coffee. So, changing a few habits throughout the day can perhaps lessen some of the severity of multiple variables.

Within the Pain Scale most people will hover around the "Breaking Point". Often only an emergency will get us into a mindset that we need to get something fixed or taken care of. Then when these people do get help they will stop suddenly when the pain is gone. So, if you look at the Pain Scale and stop right after the pain has disappeared you have just gone a hair below the breaking point. Sure, you can't feel any pain, however, you have not taken care of the trauma around the

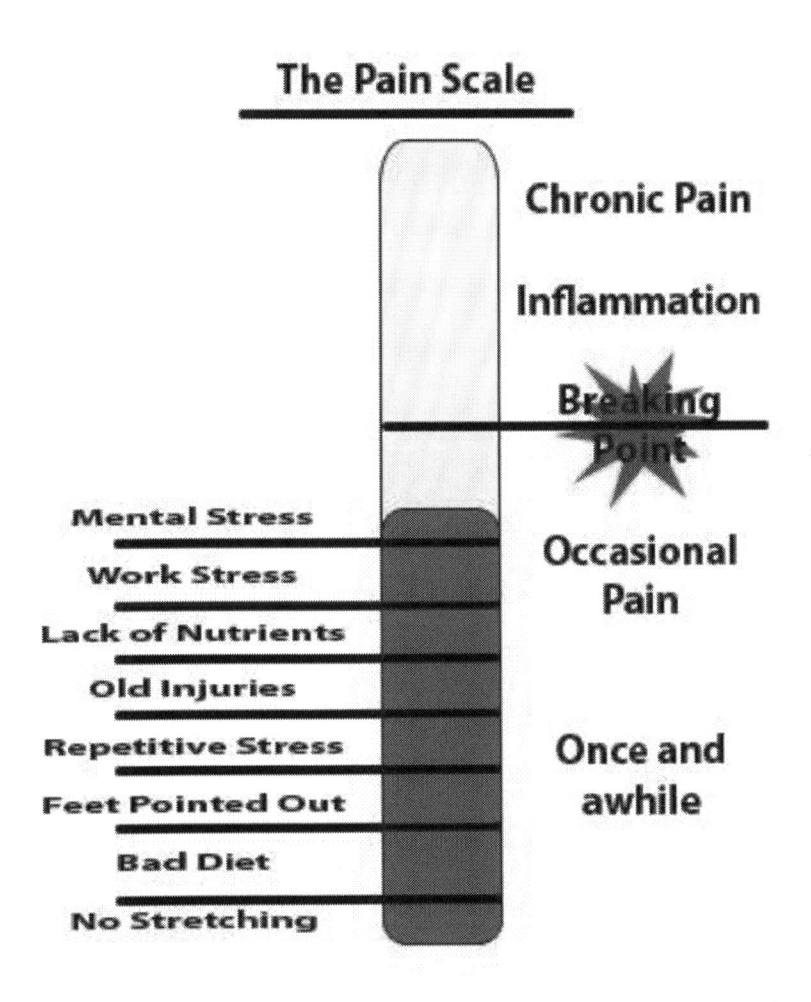

The Pain Scale

Chronic Pain

Inflammation

Breaking Point

Occasional Pain

Once and awhile

- Mental Stress
- Work Stress
- Lack of Nutrients
- Old Injuries
- Repetitive Stress
- Feet Pointed Out
- Bad Diet
- No Stretching

injured area. Your former injured soft tissue could still be weak. At this point this is where you can do firmer therapies like deep tissue massage. Workouts that focus on strengthening balance and enforcing better posture. Getting treatments while not in pain is great. You can work on the rest of your body and not have to focus on only one part of your body. When you keep your body flexible and strong you will have more tolerance to deal with more stressful situations. Just being content to hover around the breaking point means in one strange step you can reinjure yourself or worse.

Pain Scale – Optimum Range

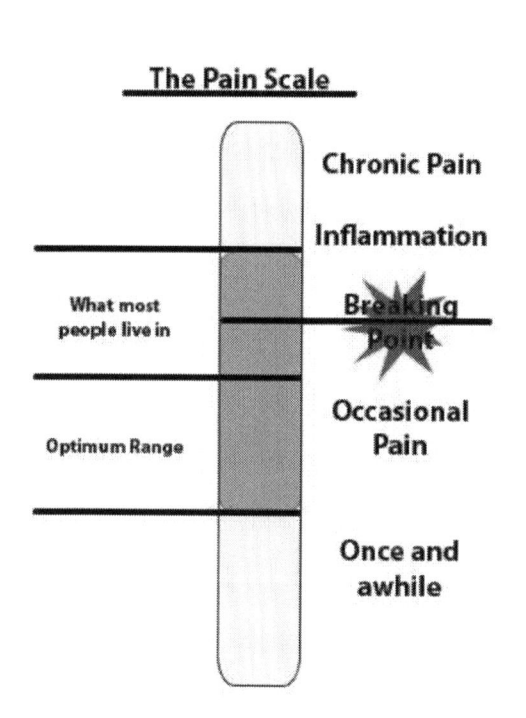

The Pain Scale

Chronic Pain

Inflammation

What most people live in

Breaking Point

Occasional Pain

Optimum Range

Once and awhile

After your injury has healed and you have been doing some therapeutic work, keep going and get yourself into the Optimal Range of the Pain Scale. The Optimal Range requires being diligent and consistent with your body to prevent injury, strengthen old injuries, and keep yourself pliable and bendable. So, if you do injure yourself again it will be less severe, and you will recover faster.

Muscle Pull Injury

Regarding the Pain Scale. It shows where our body has a breaking point. The body can take some abuse but when it tries to tell you when it is about to break, and you ignore it, it will sit you down with a mandatory time out like a pulled muscle. A pulled muscle will take 1-2 weeks to recover from. If you have hurt yourself and you are moving like a robot, you have pulled a muscle. Often a pulled muscle is a muscle that is already overstretched, and it has hardened. Then when you pull it further is when you have partially torn it and/or stretched the nerve. This is very inflammatory and the body "puffs up". This event is a warning from the body. It is telling you that if you pull this any farther you are going to rip the muscle off the bone. The body is asking for pliability, rest, and proper alignment.

When looking at the pain scale there are various levels of pain. The more out of balance we are and the more we ignore the warning signs the more painful things are. Each injury and joint imbalance add up over time. You may not feel any of this until it is too late. The body doesn't want to tell you everything that is wrong otherwise you will get nothing done. So, even if you have had an injury and have gotten some treatment and now the pain is gone; it is important to keep receiving therapy treatment to that area. Even though the injury has gone below the level of exuding no pain, it still needs some attention to strengthen. Within an injury it will hardened or create scar tissue to quickly protect itself. So, it needs to expand and be flexed. Circulation is one of the main attributes of healing. Flexing a muscle will produce circulation by exiting the old damaged cells and bringing in new nutrients for muscle repair.

So, it is good to know where you have been injured. It may be a constant exercise to know where your injuries are as they are more likely to tighten up first over time. They may need to be constantly exercised to maintain pliability. If you are constantly reinjuring yourself it may be because you have stopped your therapy right at the "no pain" line or you have not strengthened it enough to move it further down the Pain Scale.

Fatigue and repetitive motion even with perfect technique can create issues as well. That is why rest and preventable therapy will help you achieve this balance. When you overwork a muscle, it needs to repair. If you do not rest or repair it enough, it will slowly work against you

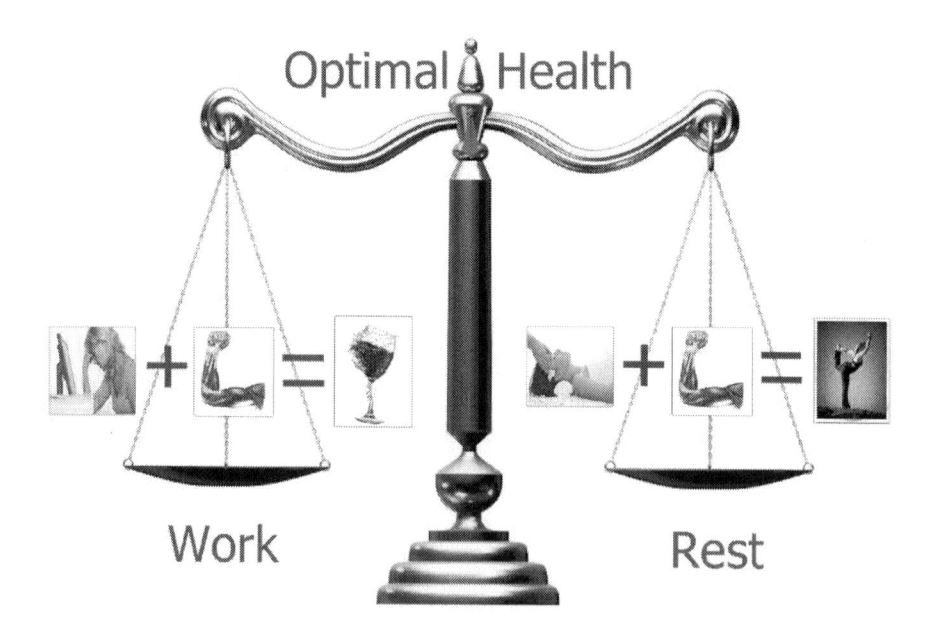

Optimal Health

Work   Rest

and become weakened. Make sure to reach the proper balance of work and rest.

Old Injuries

If an old injury is not treated or was not treated enough, it can create scar tissue. The muscle will still be stuck in the position it was injured in. This will limit the movement of the muscle and will affect the range of motion of the joint. If the joint is taken in a different direction or in a sudden manner this can create microtearing of that muscle creating more inflammation. It's Imperative to repair your injuries, keep joints mobile, hydrate so muscles can be fluid. Otherwise an old injury can resurface and become a bigger problem later.

If you have been injured, it is likely that you will have to take care of this injury for the rest of your life. We must know where our injuries are and continually keep them moving and strong. An injury can compromise ligaments and stretch things out of place or scar tissue will shorten the length of the muscle which can minimize some of its flexibility.

I like to think of recovering from old injuries is like reforming plastic. You must keep working them to reshape them back into place. If an old injury has been there awhile the rest of your body may be out of place due to forming with it or it has settled into a compromising posture.

I like the analogy of reforming your injuries is like forging a sword. First the blacksmith will heat up the fire and then use a hammer and anvil to shape the sword, continual reshaping and firing will continue to transform the shape of the sword. Afterwards the sword is dipped in cold water to be set in place. A form of this can be copied by hot tubbing, heat pads, or stretching to warm up the area. Then do some flexing of the muscle to break up the scar tissue and flex your muscles into place. Then rest or ice the area.

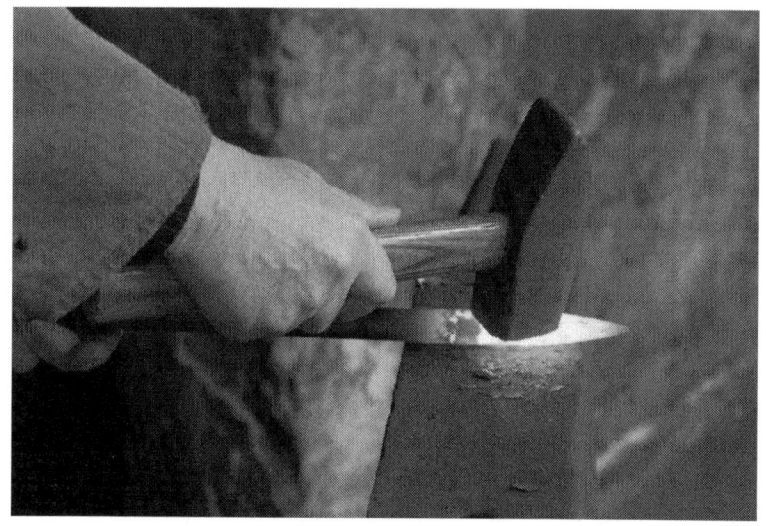

https://pixabay.com/en/forge-craft-hot-form-iron-550622/

Motion does not create Pain?

I go on with these points because there is a faction of people who believe that motion does not create pain. I am making the case that there are a variety of ways to create pain and there is no absolute way to compare people's issues exactly together. That is why there will likely never be one pill that solves everything or one stretch that will resolve everything.

Many of these people point to experiments such as this one.

https://www.ncbi.nlm.nih.gov/pubmed/2951745

https://www.sciencedirect.com/science/article/pii/S0021929017303135

https://www.jospt.org/doi/abs/10.2519/jospt.2017.7268?code=jospt-site

They take people with low back pain and see that they have a tilt in their pelvis. They take another group with no back pain and tilt their pelvis in the same manner. The conclusion is that the 2nd group has no back pain so therefore pain is not caused by motion.

Then there was this study that was pointed out to me with the experiment of 67 people who had scapular dyskinesis. Which is chronic inflammation from moving the shoulder in a particular motion. The 67 demonstrated what action of their shoulder that pain was caused in. Then they used 68 people who did not have shoulder pain. Put them through the same movements as the 67. The 68 people without pain did not have pain when their shoulder was in the same position. Therefore, this data is being used for people to say that posture does not create pain.[27]

It is impossible to replicate this experiment with humans as there are so many different things that we do. If the back pain was created due to 10 years of sitting with their toes pointed out. The only experiment to prove this is the 2nd group would need to sit in the same chair, the same way, for 10 years. Then we add in stress, meditation, nutrition and all the other variables and there is really no way to find an absolute one-cause situation to any issue. I am making the case that there is a variety of issues that come together and without proper maintenance in a timely way these issues will compound and manifest. Seems people want to have an absolute reason for something and if it is not absolute then it is not useful data and then things on the contrary are absolutely debunked.

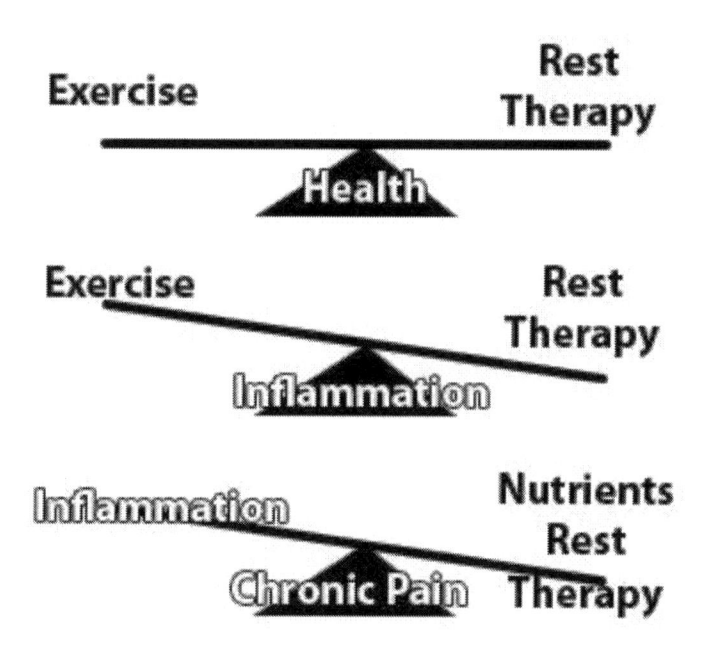

```
        Exercise              Rest
                              Therapy
        ─────────────────────────────
                    ▲Health

        Exercise              Rest
                              Therapy
        ─────────────────────────────
                ▲Inflammation

        Inflammation      Nutrients
                          Rest
        ─────────────────────────────
                ▲Chronic Pain  Therapy
```

Balancing Work vs Therapy

Balance is the key to life which is harmony and ultimate health. We need to move and exercise. When we do exercise, things break down and we need to rest. There is a constant breathe in and breathe out, flex this way then flex the other. When the scales become weighted in one direction more than the other we create imbalance. Things fatigue faster and break down quicker.

When we do enough exercise and do the appropriate rest and therapy we have health. When we do not do enough rest, we start to accumulate injuries and then create inflammation. If we ignore this accumulation, we move up the Pain Scale and create chronic pain which seems to have no resolution. When we have balance we have peace and health.

So, it is imperative to use this walking naturally method to align your muscles, keep joints loose, keep pumping synovial fluid, stay hydrated, flex your muscle groups in both directions, proper supporting nutrition, and rest. When we have too many of these variables out of balance this may be the cause to how osteoarthritis is created. When we can get some of these levels balanced and moving it may be possible to prevent and hopefully resolve osteoarthritis.

Chapter Eleven

Mental Manifesting

"All truly great thoughts are conceived while walking."
— **Friedrich Nietzsche, <u>Twilight of the Idols</u>**

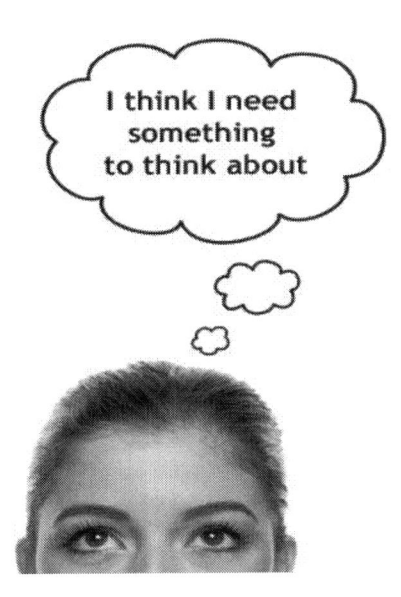

As a Medical Intuitive, I have learned that the source of pain and disease starts in your mental interpretation of the world. The body's health is the direct result and reflection of your Mind's health. When the mind decides to create something, there is a specific process that happens from the initial identification of a problem all the way to a physical manifestation that remedies the situation. The same thing can be said about the technique of throwing a ball. If there is a problem with the throwing action somewhere, in the mind will be the same problem. A walking stride can exhibit the same pattern as the mind process. If one has a hiccup in the mind, the body will copy and express the same hiccup. So, pain and circumstance can reflect the same pattern you may be skipping in your mental manifestations.

In the "Four Step Points" Chapter, I go into the specifics of the Four Step Points for the physical body. Really, I should start with the Mental Aspects of walking before the Physical aspects of walking. However, not a lot of people are ready to hear about the concept that they may be causing their own health demise. Also, if you want to put your health back on your terms, you are going to have to do your own research. I recommend getting multiple opinions from practitioners from different modalities. With the myriad of opinions, I read between the lines and choose what I am going to do. People would rather blame others and genetics for their health problems. I can confidently tell you from my experience it does hurt at first, but if you can accept this concept, that you create your health, then you will see so many life improvements occur. When you take responsibility for your own health, your life will go from boring and hopeless to purposeful and joyful. Putting all your faith in others exposes you to be a victim of your own ignorance.

By being able to observe how my body works, I have also been able to observe how my mind works and I have come up with these 4 Mental Step Points that correspond to the 4 Physical Step Points.

The 4 Mental Step Points:

1. Clear intention of dreams and desires.[1]
2. Commit to Action.[2]
3. Following Through.[3]
4. Accepting the Outcome.[4]

Steps 1 & 2 both work with developing a clear plan and then deciding to fulfill it, as it relates to current wants and needs. Steps 3-4 work with the "doing" of said intention and being responsible to see the plan and accepting the good with the bad. Once this action is complete, reflection upon the outcome will determine what needs to be done for next time.

Both techniques of the spiritual mind connecting with the body are crucial factors that must be looked at. Using one or the other is not enough. The sum will be added up in our overall physical and spiritual health. Every issue can be resolved if we focus on the physical symptoms and the mental issues. If the mind is the source of the pain, just taking care of the body may delay resolutions and the issue will come up again later.

Ideally, it is best to work with a variety of practitioners who work in different areas. A spiritual advisor or counselor is best for Spiritual and Mental guidance and on the physical level, herbs and manual therapies are also helpful. When you witness how each practitioner solves your issues then you can see the bigger part of the equation. If you only work with one practitioner or modality, then you may only see a small part of the big picture which may not make any sense.

In the Chapter "Toes Forward" - 80% of the People walk with their toes outward and then there is the 20% of people walk with their toes inward.

The Mental Aspect of the 80% outward toe walkers

I have noticed a pattern within each group in their Mental Step Points. When you walk with your toes outward you will roll Step Points 3 & 4 together at the same time. Specifically, Step Point 4 is being skipped. This point must do with "Accepting the Outcome". When you have your toes pointed outward this means you really don't want to "get there". Sometimes when we find out we have been doing something wrong we go into denial and don't want to hear that we have been sabotaging a piece of ourselves for most of our life. It takes a lot of courage to be able to hear constructive criticism without becoming upset and taking it personally. What we should really be putting into our intention is, "I want to be the best at what I do, so I will listen to all possible aspects that I may be doing wrong." When you can listen to a coach or counselor giving you advice to improve your performance this will only enhance the outcome. The same goes with running a business, completing a project, or listening to your partner. By being open to hear guidance from others and hear the painful advice from your body, this will be the beginning of putting you on track for optimal health on your terms. Understanding how things truly work and then implementing them is the grand key to achieving enlightenment, soul purpose, and pure bliss.

The Mental Aspect of the 20% inward toe walkers

The other 20% that walk with their toes pointed inwards are skipping Step Points 1 & 2. They are running on their toes and not hitting the heel. These people are usually in a big rush and are always falling forward. Because they have not clearly stated their goals on what they specifically want, they have the feeling of always being behind. When you don't state your goals then you do a lot of extra running around hoping you run into them. They are also in such a rush and they will always overlook the opportunity because it has not manifested yet. One must be patient and allow your intention to manifest. It is a lot like throwing a ball; these people will throw the ball of intention and then expend all their energy to run to where the ball is landing. Then they get hit in the back of the head and they think that next time they just need to run faster. In fact, all they need to do is trust that they are playing catch with the universe and are supposed to throw the ball and let the universe throwback something better in return.

Inward toe walkers need to let that heel dig into the ground and SLOW DOWN. Be patient with where you are at because chasing your tail ends up in the same place that you started. Watch and you will see that by slowing down you will get more things done and will waste way less time and resources.

So instead of slamming the door on the unwanted house guest called pain, invite it in as a secret counsel for the next steps you need to take. Empowering ourselves and being responsible for our own lives brings clarity and purpose to living. We are shown everyday hints on how to lead our lives and pain is one those gifts. Embrace the messenger and walk in peace.

Chapter Twelve

Shoes - The Good, Bad, and the Funny Looking

"But the beauty is in the walking -- we are betrayed by destinations." ─ **Gwyn Thomas**

Bad Shoes

As previously stated in the "Gripping the Ground Chapter", it is best to be able to feel the ground and fully flex your feet. In the waitress world, there is a popular shoe that most wear that is like a clog. The sole is very hard, and the foot cannot flex into the ground. Many waitresses and servers have low back, hip, or leg issues. When waitresses change their shoes to a more flexible shoe, their issues cease within a week. Binding your feet or wearing too cushy of a sole does not help foot health either. Flexing and actively stretching your feet is best for circulation and structure strengthening.[1]

Ideal Shoes

I like to wear Skechers, which are in my opinion, a sporty good-looking shoe. The sole is very thin, and I can really feel the ground. Another Shoe company with a thin sole is Vibram, I like to call their shoes "Monkey Feet", and they look like gloves for your feet. This is the best shoe scenario because one will ultimately feel every piece of the ground and your feet will become very strong. However, one must start out slow because walking correctly at first is very hard because you are accentuating muscles that you have not used in a while. When you start to use these new muscles, they will fatigue quickly. So, pace yourself and work the walking technique slowly.

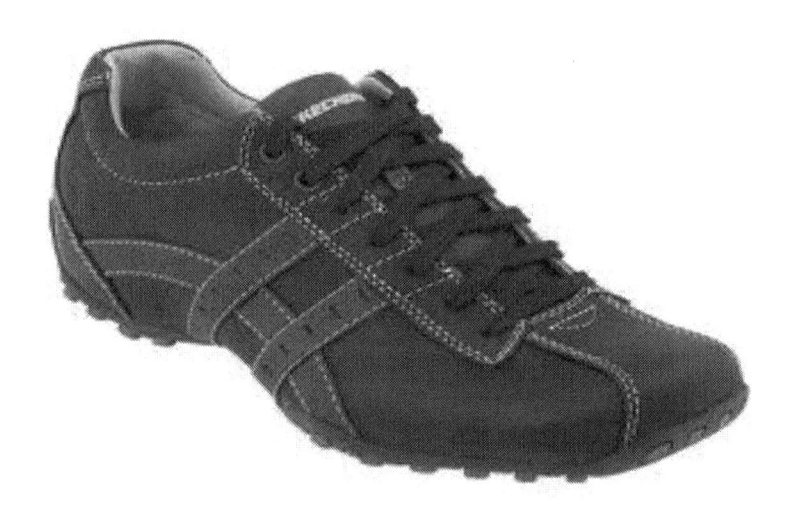

www.skechers.com

New Shoes

If you are going to start walking naturally, you are going to want to get some new shoes. Attempting to walk naturally with your old shoes that are worn out is very difficult. As the shoes wear out naturally the wear will continually get worse and your walking technique also gets slowly worse. If you walk on the outside of your feet, the heel and outside edge becomes more and more worn and attempting to hit the inside foot becomes harder to do. It feels like you have a large bump in your shoe which makes walking naturally harder to maintain. Try this walking naturally technique in new shoes for a while and then put your old shoes back on. You will then see a big difference.

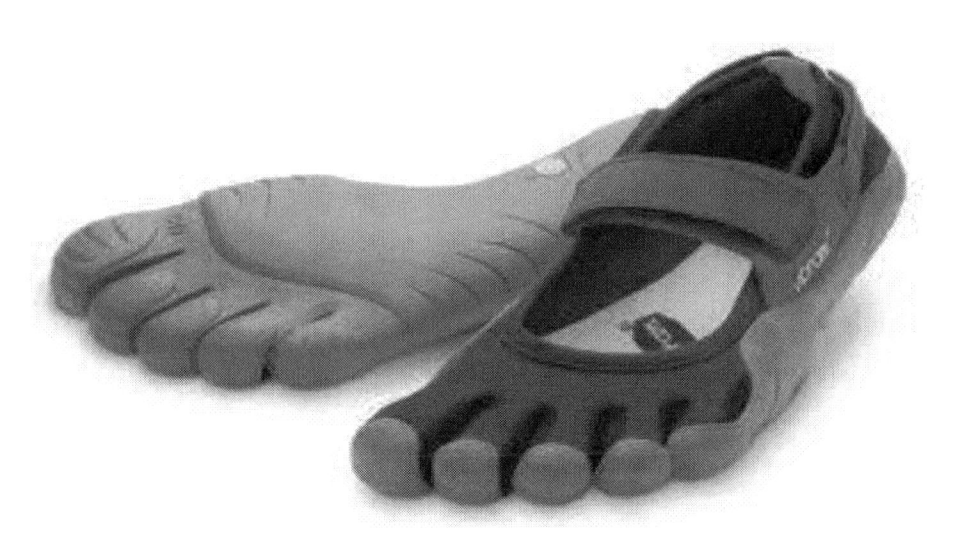

- www.us.vibram.com

Ladies in Heels

Do I really need to bother? Heels are only for getting your picture taken. Once the picture is taken then change into some flats. Heels focus too much of the weight into the front of the feet. Also, they will make your hamstrings very tight. Ankles will have too much pressure on them and forget about being able to flex the arch of your foot.[2]

I have been able to observe my shoes lasting much longer now because I work my feet evenly on both sides. So not only will walking naturally help your leg joint health but will also help you from buying more shoes.

Tip: Walking barefoot over rocks is a fantastic way to massage and strengthen your feet.

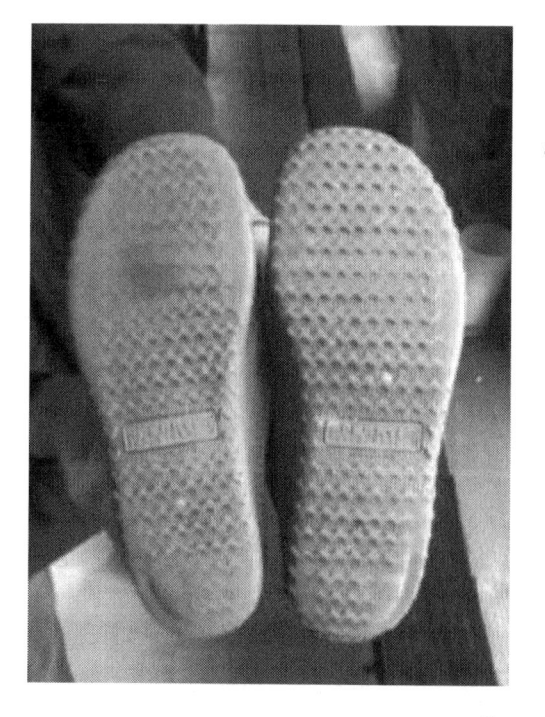

Note the worn tread from leaning to the right side while walking. Also see the bottom outside heels are worn from pointing the toes outward.

Chapter Thirteen

Sports and Recreation

Between professional sports and recreational activities technique plays a part. In higher level competitions, races are lost and won by thousandths of a second which can be the difference of a nose length. If two competitors of equal strength were racing and one had poor technique and the other had good technique, it is likely good technique will win out. The other important factor is that the good technique athlete will likely have less wear and tear on their body and if injured they will repair faster. In recreation sports winning may not be important but the thrill and exercise component is what is desired. No one likes being injured so whether you are on a bike or a snowboard, leg technique is important to preventing injuries or trying to recover from an old injury.

Biking

In the Chapter of "Toes Forward", it was discussed on the importance of having your toes pointed forward while walking. When they are pointed outward we can create low back pain. In biking it is important to watch the position of your knees and that they do not point outward. This means you are not using your inside leg muscles. This may also mean you are pushing on the pedals with the outside edges of your feet, which is associated with shin splints. On machines like bikes, ellipticals, rowing machines, tread mills it is easy to cheat technique because you are moving a machine and not your body.

On a bike you want your knees pointed forward, this will engage your inner legs more. This will also evenly disperse the weight on both sides of your feet. When you bring your knees in, when your leg is behind you while peddling, you should be accessing the inside leg muscles

Riding a Bike

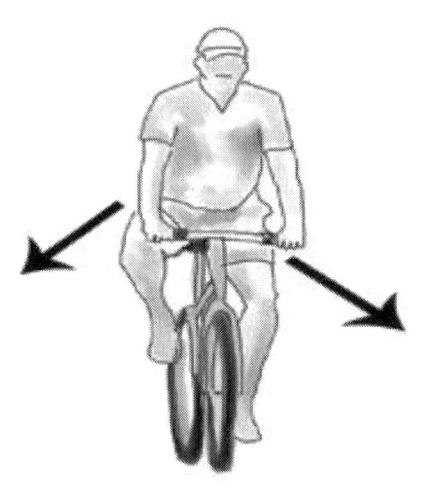

Make sure your knees are pointed forward. When they are pointed outward you will not be accessing your inside leg muscles.

and when your foot is in front of you, you are using your outside leg muscles.

Snowboarding

Even though your feet may be strapped to a board and things may seem immovable. I have noticed while snowboarding that when leaning you are using your leg muscles. In the "Toes Forward" Chapter it is discussed if you have your feet pointed inwards you will fall

Snowboarding Slalom

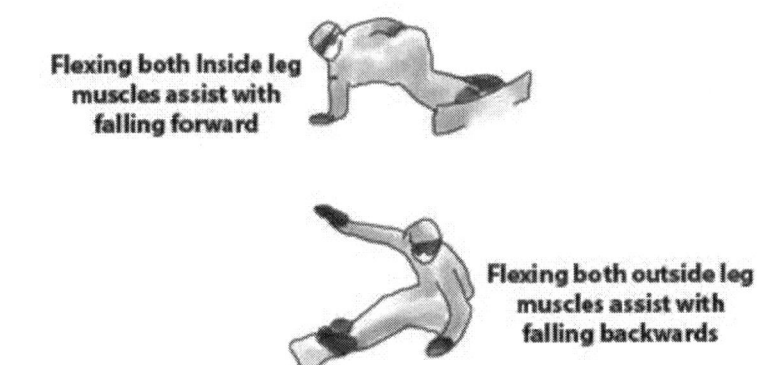

Flexing both Inside leg muscles assist with falling forward

Flexing both outside leg muscles assist with falling backwards

Important to maintain linking the core muscles to the feet on both the inner and outer leg muscles.

forward. If you have your feet turned out, you will fall backwards. While slaloming down a hill you are doing this. If you have your left foot forward and turning to the right, you will be using your inside legs to help you fall forward to take a turn. When turning left in the middle of the turn you lean on your outside leg muscles to fall backwards. So, when turning right you use your inner core and inside leg muscles to make the turn. When turning left you are using your outside leg muscles and lower back. Of course, things are reversed for the right foot forward crowd.

Skating

Outdoor and Indoor Skating

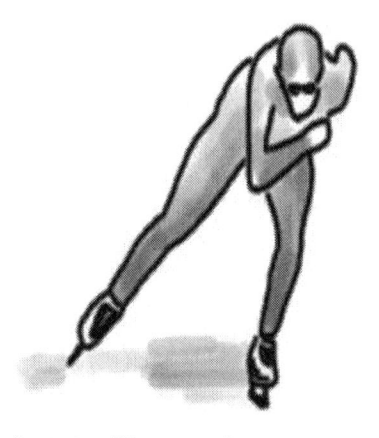

Important if in a sport that goes in the same direction like a track, to make sure to cross-train and go the other direction. This will assist in even muscle development and prevent injuries.

Whether it's ice skating or roller skating these sports require a lot of inside leg muscles. To move forward is about pushing off your inside leg. Make sure to engage your core with your inside leg muscles.

A repeating theme in this book is if you are going to flex one way make sure to flex the other way. So those sports that involve a track like short track ice skating or indoor roller skating. They are often turning left only. This can develop into injuries in the groin, ankle's and knees.[1]

I urge these people to spend 50% of the practice turning left and the other 50% of the practice turning right as you go around the track. Sure, you must practice turning left but what you are also doing is overdeveloping muscles in one direction over a period. If we can exercise those muscles in the other direction I believe there will be less ankle and knee injuries associated with the sport. You can cheat technique when you have youth on your side, but if you want to compete at the highest levels longer than most; it is imperative to have a technique that helps you rather than hurts you. Then you will have a longer career and recreationally you can extend your sport into your older years.

Skiing

Skiing of course requires a lot of leg strength. One can be going very fast down a hill and when your have both legs strapped to two different devices things can easily go wrong. Knee issues are a common issue for skiing, one specific condition that can be compromised is the Medial Collateral Ligament (MCL). This happens when the knee is bent, and a force hits the outside of the knee. This can happen while falling or in my opinion, this can be a gradual injury due to people not supporting or flexing their inside leg muscles.[2]

To help prevent this injury it is important to be strong between both of your inner legs. In the "Falling Arches" Chapter, we talked about holding the bridge or arch of your foot. The same thing can be said about the arch of your legs. If you draw a line from inner leg to your core down the other inner leg this is an arch. It is important to maintain this arch while sloming.

Catching an edge in skiing can be common. This is when you want to take a turn and your body goes one way but one of your skis does not

Ski Slalom

Inside Leg Muscles

Outside Leg Muscles

**Important to link the abdominal core to the inside leg muscles.
Maintain the arch of the core to the bottom of the inside foot.**

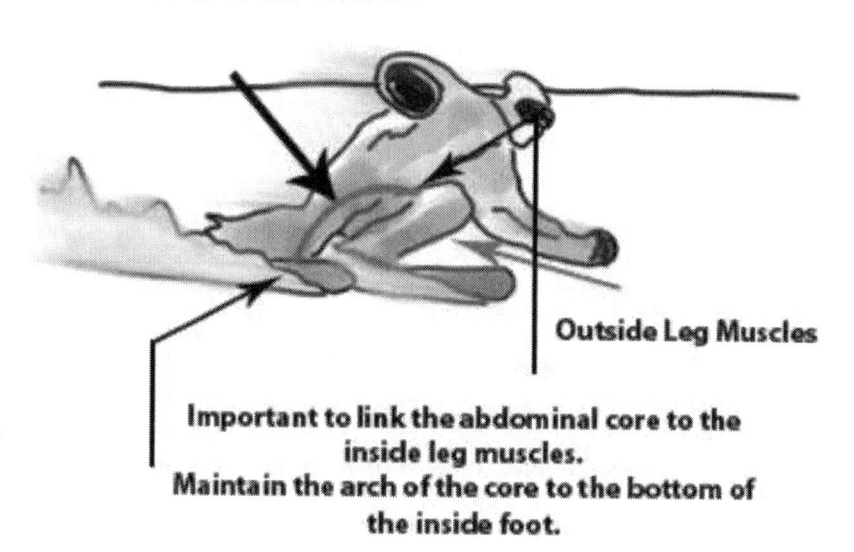

bite into the snow and then it goes the opposite way. This is one way to twist an ankle or a knee.

So being strong with your inner legs will help support slaloming. If you are going down hill and turning left, with your right leg you are using your inside leg muscles. Your left leg will be using the outside leg muscles. Then when your turn right, your right leg will use the outside leg muscles and your left leg will flex the inside leg muscles. The inner legs are associated with activating the core. It is likely you are using your core the whole way down the hill to assist with turning. Being aware of this posture will help in protecting your knees if you fall or catch an edge.

The core will also help in stabilizing the torso. You don't want your torso flailing around while turning. You want your torso locked in with your core. The main thing to focus on is the arch of the inner legs and your torso should be inline with it. One must be strong with the inner legs and this will help with balance and supporting your knees. This will also help you in maintaining strong turns and letting the skis do the work not your upper body.

Later in the book I talk about the yoga position of the chair pose. It is about strengthening the inner legs. When you take an object like a ball and place it between your knees, then strike the chair pose. This will help to strengthen the arch of your inner legs. To take it a step further, sway back and forth like you are sloaming. This will help to strengthen the tiny muscles in your feet and knees that are used for balancing.

Football and Repeating Injuries

If you are continually injuring a body part this is a clue of bad technique. Within sports your body must bend in awkward positions sometimes to get a ball or maneuver over a jump. Often when things go wrong is when we hurt ourselves. I would like to focus more on how bad technique creates injuries. Often, in an awkward fall or impact we will get injured in an area that is already weakened due to bad technique. But then we just blame it on the event of the fall.

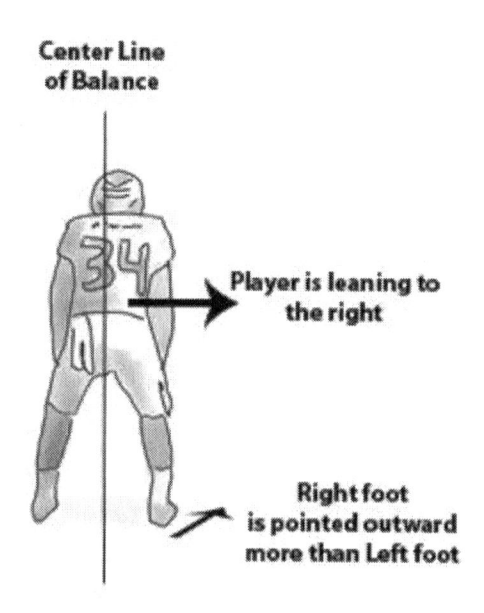

Center Line of Balance

Player is leaning to the right

Right foot is pointed outward more than Left foot

Player #34 is a Running Back. A year before this picture his lower right leg was broken. He is still running around "injuried".

Watching some football players, they are involved in a lot of impact tackles. However, when I watch them walk to the sideline they have their feet pointed outward, like a lot of people. Then you throw in some tackles and this will exasperate things. It is almost like the what came first the chicken or the egg? In football what came first, the impact or were they already walking in away that was not supporting their legs. I of course believe it is both. You can't prevent the impact, but you can prevent your body from getting as injured and recover quicker if you walk in away that supports good walking technique.

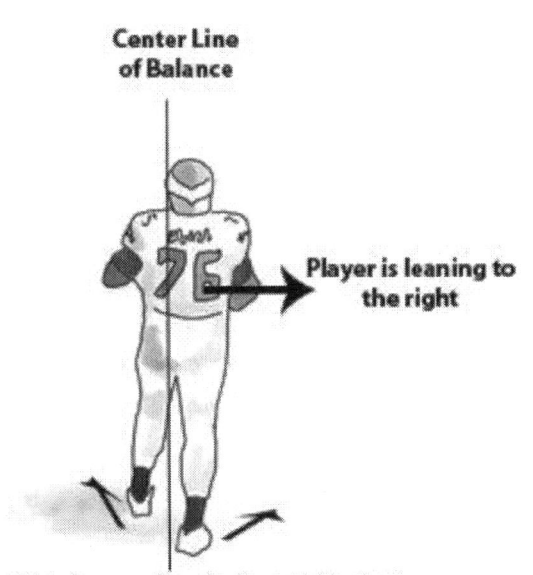

Center Line of Balance

Player is leaning to the right

#76 had a very bad injury to his right knee. The effects of walking on his right side are still there 2 years later.

135

A common injury a hear is hamstrings, groins, or low back issues. If a football player has one of these it is likely to come back and be an ongoing issue with them. These issues are due to having your feet pointed outwards. When you walk like this the weight of your body is centered on the back end of your legs and therefore you will have tight hamstrings. This will also mean you are over stretching your inside leg muscles creating a potential groin pull. This will make the outside leg muscles tight compromising the knees which will also directly affect the low back.

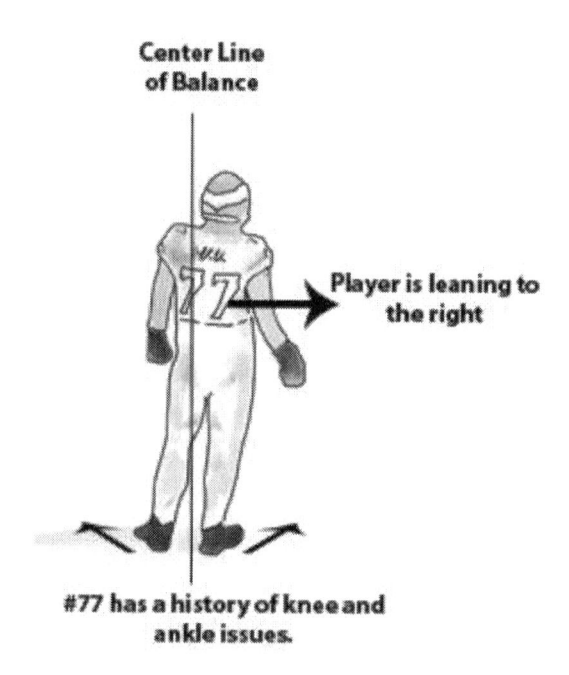

Center Line of Balance

Player is leaning to the right

#77 has a history of knee and ankle issues.

If a football player or anyone in the running sports has a problem with one of these issues they may soon have another one of these symptoms. Plantar fasciitis will quickly come because if you have an injury to your leg, your ankle will lock up to prevent further injury. Then all joints will lock up on the same leg from the ankle, knee, and hip. It is important to let the injury rest and heal. If you injured one leg you may be walking on the other for a while as well.

#89 is having repeating leg injuries, from Groin, Hamstring, and Knee issues. These issues are associated with feet pointed outwards.

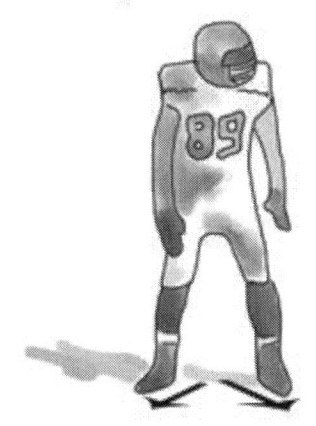

Both Feet are constantly pointed outwards

Once it has healed you want to start with exercising the axis of opening and closing of the foot. Make sure to distribute your weight evenly on both legs. I have seen many people who have been injured over a decade or two ago and they are still walking around on one leg like they are still injured. And of course, they will have an additional leg or back injury due to walking around like they are still injured. If you are injured, you need to know which way you were injured and over emphasize what good technique is. When injured we walk around compromising our bodies for sometimes months. This then becomes

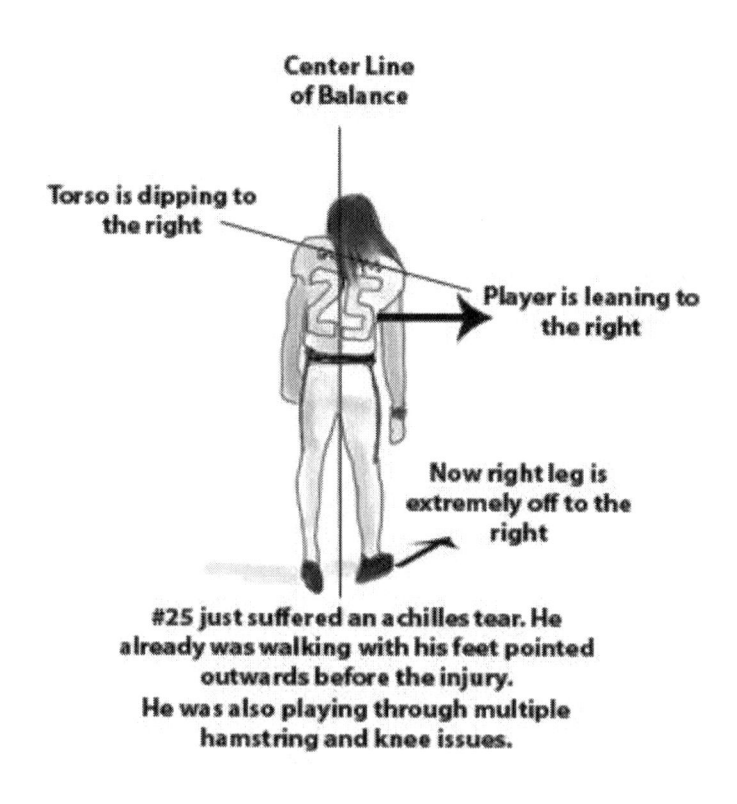

Center Line of Balance

Torso is dipping to the right

Player is leaning to the right

Now right leg is extremely off to the right

#25 just suffered an achilles tear. He already was walking with his feet pointed outwards before the injury.
He was also playing through multiple hamstring and knee issues.

a habit and even though the pain is gone we are still walking around on one leg or not flexing our foot properly.

Football players have a short season, so they don't want to be out for too long. What would assist in a speedier recovery and hope of not having a reoccurring injury is to practice walking with good technique. Walking incorrectly with your toes outward may not cause an injury. However, because you are compromising your joints by having them pointed in one direction all the time, when it comes to a compromising position the integrity of the joint or muscle may be easily injured. If the injured player would walk with good technique, they would recover faster and would be less prone to reinjury. When we walk in a way that does not compromise our body, it will focus on healing. However, if the player does not walk with more of a conscious technique, the injury will not heal as quickly. This may result in an ongoing cascade of injuries that are all related. If a knee has been injured, then it is easy for a hip or ankle injury to happen next.[3]

Chapter Fourteen

Therapies, Solutions, & Exercises for Superior Walking Health

"Everywhere is walking distance if you have the time."
— **Steven Wright**

Walking Meditation – Grounding to the Earth

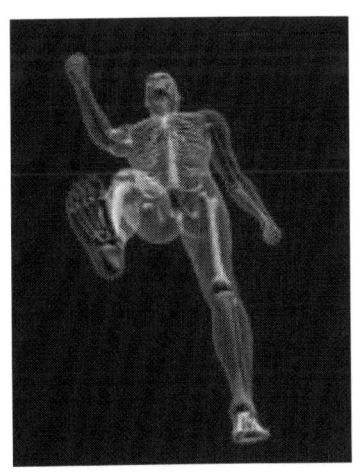

For all those over-thinkers who can't get out of their head, thinking about your feet is a great meditation exercise. Often the term used for this is called "Grounding" or "Grounding to the Earth". When one thinks about how their feet touches the ground, it helps you forget about repetitive or useless thoughts. This is another habit to break. The addiction of worrying about things that will never happen. When you are in your head worrying about such things you are not thinking about the position or posture of your body. Letting go of mental stress and thinking about how your body moves through space in a calm manner is a meditation. When you do begin to ground to the earth it's like you are pulling all the excess thoughts out of your head and using it as glue to connect with the Earth. If you really think about it, with all that thinking, do you really get more done? Taking a break and feeling your body touch the earth, will help your conscious rest and your subconscious will come up with better ideas. Plus, when you take time to rest your body, the mind has a better house to settle in.

Ultimately walking naturally will help prevent most of these self-inflicted issues and will help in strengthening and exercising injuries of the past. However, receiving some manual therapies will help in relieving a lot of these issues such as chiropractic, acupuncture, and massage. However, at the end of the day you can get all the treatment you want but if your pain is self-inflicted from your daily routine you may never completely resolve your pain. You can think that just because you are getting therapy, that will be the end, and you don't have to do anything yourself.

One of the best times to walk correctly is after you have received a body work session. When you are calm from a massage or your bones have been aligned due to a chiropractic session, this is the best time to practice walking naturally and get your body to be familiar with what it is like to walk correctly when things are aligned. Trying to walk naturally while compromised due to tight injuries and bad posture that is cemented in the wrong position is the slow road to recovery.

I believe it is best to receive a variety of treatments from different practitioners. Each practitioner and modality will have a different opinion about the same issue. It is up to you to be the master of your bodies domain and read between the lines of the different suggestions from your therapists. When practitioners start saying things that are similar that is information to listen to. There are varying ideas on how to use an ice pack. Some say 10 minutes, others will say 30 minutes, in this case I shoot for the average and will go for 20 minutes. But ultimately, you need to take all these things as suggestions and monitor yourself. If it feels good to you and your injury is improving, then stick with that.

Often with swelling it may take 2-3 days for the swelling to kick in and then people forget how they got injured because of something they did 3 days ago. We must think broader with health and recovery is a slow long-term game. In this society we want things instant and now. When it comes to healing we need to do things slow and when we do, true recovery will happen.

I have seen a pattern with injuries. Usually things happen when people are not paying attention, stressed out, or in a rush. Often this is when we get injured. So, when you are forcibly sidelined I like to think of this time as a reminder to slow down and rethink how you are doing things. The injury may be a sign from the Universe or your inner self to slow things down so that you can get things right.

Chiropractors

Chiropractors manage the spinal system. Their hands-on therapy can correct vertebra that is out of place. When nerves are compressed in the spine this can lead to constant back pain and it can also compromise organ health as specific nerves go from the spine to specific organs.[1]

When we are injured in a car accident or sport injury our bodies may stay stuck in the position we fell into or our bodies were whiplashed and forced into position we don't normally are in. Muscles will be in trauma and they will hold and pull the muscles out of place. When bones are put back into place the muscles will calm down.

A 2010 study published in the *Journal of Manipulative Physiological Therapies* found that nearly 60 percent of patients with sciatica who failed other medical treatments benefited from spinal manipulation just as well as if they had undergone surgical intervention! [2]

Trying these kinds of therapies is a good place to start. Surgery should be looked as a last resort.

One study published in the *Official Journal of the North American Spinal Society* found that after comparing results in 102 adults who suffered from sciatic nerve pain, those who received chiropractic adjustments experienced less local pain, fewer number of days with pain, and fewer cases of moderate or severe pain compared to people who didn't receive adjustments.[3]

Acupuncture

Acupuncture is about opening the bodies natural flow of energy. It uses needles to target specific paths/meridians to move energy throughout the body. Swelling can block circulation which will also compromise the flow of energy. This stuck energy can cause pain. The pain is signaling that the body needs some circulation. Circulation helps move old cellular debris out and bring healing nutrients in. Acupuncture is a good modality to integrate with massage and chiropractic.

If you can't stand needles there are alternate therapies that Acupuncturists use like needleless acupuncture, TENS Units, Tuning Forks, and Shiatsu.[4]

Massage Therapy

Massage is great for loosening very tight walking muscles. When you have been walking for decades incorrectly it is difficult to just go cold turkey and suddenly start successfully walking the correct way. Improper technique has become a habit and breaking habits takes some time to undo. After decades of walking incorrectly, overstretched muscles can be very difficult to engage. Overstretched muscles will usually be the muscles that are causing the pain. Flexing these muscles will keep them from becoming more stretched and once flexed they will stretch the over used tight muscles which exhibit no pain. "Typical toe outward" people will have tight outside legs and overstretched inside legs.[5]

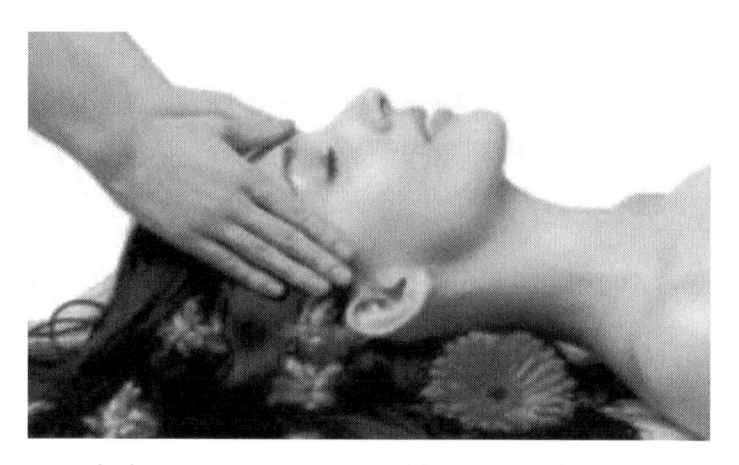

Massage can help get you started walking correctly because massage techniques such as cross fiber friction can help break up scar tissue in the muscles. Once these tight muscles can relax a bit it will be easier to flex and strengthen the overstretched muscles. "Knots" and "ropey" muscles are overstretched muscles. They have become this way because when a muscle is overstretched, it must protect itself by hardening. The overstretched muscles are the ones that exude the pain because the tendon is about to be ripped from the bone. Tight muscles are the real cause which usually exudes no pain because they are stealing the space from the overstretched muscles. It is like a tug a war in your body. The best way to resolve the battle is to balance the scale. Flex overstretched muscles and stretch the tight ones. You can rub overstretched muscles all day and it will have very little lasting effect. By stretching and lengthening the tight muscle that gives off no pain, you will have more beneficial relief to the overstretched muscle.

Yoga: Chair Pose

Studies have found that yoga is safe and effective for people with sciatic nerve pain. Some of the most important movements for preventing sciatic pain target the back, building strength and relaxing stiff areas. Exercises to prevent low back pain and the core are used in rehabilitation settings for sciatic nerve patients.[6]

There are not too many exercises for the inside legs besides walking but there is one that will let you know about your inside legs. The Chair Pose!

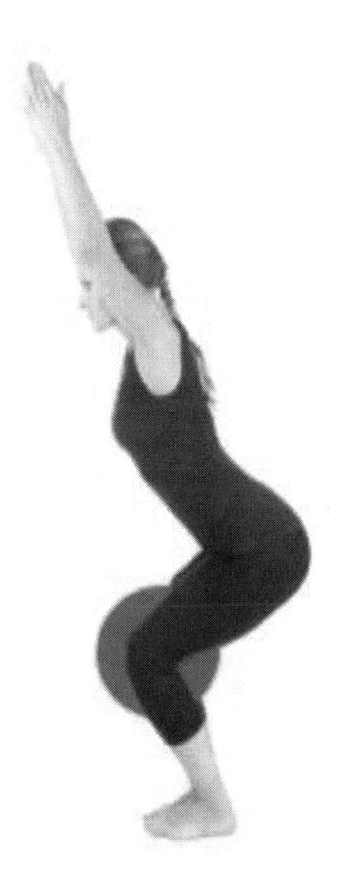

To really access the inside leg muscles, it is important to have a firm object in between your knees or thighs like a soft soccer ball, Yamana ball, firm pillow, yoga block, or a bouncy red ball.

Put the firm object between your knees and squeeze them tighter and strike the Chair Pose. Feel the inside legs burn and push your inside feet downwards into the ground.

It is important to feel these muscles as this will add more awareness to your walking technique and you will know if you are walking correctly or not.

Flexing your arch and Step Points 3 & 4 is primarily using inside leg muscles and is imperative to a correct walking posture.

Overall yoga is a great way to get your body in shape in a gentle way. It can also be an unexpected surprising workout. There are a variety of different forms of yoga. Some are meditative with gentle stretching, others a mid-level workout, and then there are very advanced poses that require a lot of balance and inner strength. I like to recommend yoga because it gets your body in different positions you would not normally get into. It strengthens joints and many of the poses focus on how you hold your body up. Yoga can be considered a form of meditation, as a lot of mindfulness is woven into the philosophy.

Another aspect I like about yoga is that you can be in a very intense and challenging pose and the practice is to relax the mind and breathe. Being in a tense situation with a reminder to breathe is a big key to dealing with stressful situations in the workplace or making crucial decisions. A lot of stress is because we are not calm when deciding. When we can give ourselves space to be calm and breathe while in a stressful state, this may lead to a better outcome and a body that is not a "brick" at the end of the day.

Prevention

Often people will be puzzled as to how this pain occurred. Some will say, "But I have been doing this for years?" I say, "That is exactly the problem, you have been doing it for years". At a certain point the body says, "No more!" If we keep ourselves in good shape and improve our flexibility in both directions of a joint; and if we repair our injuries before they get too bad, we may prevent a lot of these issues. Often people only receive therapy when it is too late, and things are broken. If you can do things like pay attention to your posture, receive therapy before things are injured, you may not need emergency therapy or be in constant pain.

Russell Wilson, Quarterback of the Seahawks receives 2 hours of massage 5 times a week. As of today, 2018 he has had some serious injuries, that have derailed some players to miss games or retire, but he has been able to recover faster and still has not missed a game or even a practice.

"I think just taking care of your body is really important, especially when you're playing in the NFL," Wilson said. "You've got to take care of yourself, stretch-up time, do everything that you can to be ready and feel your best every week. I've done that really since my rookie year, just continue to make sure I take care of my body and [am] ready to go for the game."[7]

James Harrison of the Pittsburgh Steelers is very "old" (39 in 2017) in the NFL and spends $300k on therapy to take care of his body. So, when they do get injured or put in a position where most people get hurt. These people don't get as hurt and will recover faster than their counterparts.

For his muscles to handle the lifting sessions and the NFL grind, Harrison says he needs an acupuncturist, a dry needlist, three massage therapists, two chiropractors and "a person who does cupping."[8]

"The great ones who last, it's all about recovery," said retired offensive tackle Ryan Harris, who played from 2007 to 2016. "Hydrations, IVs, meditation, yoga."[8]

I have noticed this with people who I massage who get into a car accident and their body gets whiplashed. Those that take care of themselves in a preventable manner will recover from a car accident in 1-3 months. Those that don't take care of themselves will have a recovery period of 3-12 months or longer. Being proactive in our health is one of the best things you can do to prevent chronic issues. If you have a chronic issue it is because you have waited too long and have ignored the minor warning signs. Often people get therapy when they are injured and then stop when the pain is gone. The best time to do preventative therapy is when you are not in pain. When you are not in pain and receive preventative therapy, you can go further and deeper into the body and heal those small injuries of the past. When these small injuries accumulate they may turn into a bigger more inflammatory issue.

I have found that receiving 1-2 massages a month is good for maintenance and prevention. However, if you do have an injury receiving a massage 1-2's a week will help you recover quicker.

Chapter Fifteen

What is Water?

Aside from Walking Naturally my second favorite topic I am most passionate about is water and hydration. With every person I see in my office we will at least go over the "How to Walk" or the "What is Water" lesson. If we can master these two topics, we can prevent most of the issues out there in the world.

Preventing Dehydration

When people have headaches, tight muscles, and sinus infections that linger, it is a sign of dehydration.[16] When you're properly hydrated you will rarely catch a cold or at least have one only for a day or so. If it goes on longer it is because you are dehydrated. If your nose is stuffed up it is a sign you are dehydrated. I will add a pinch of salt to a glass of water, now I have an IV. IV's are made up of water, salt, vitamins, sugar, and baking soda. Often used in the hospitals after surgery or when someone is in a health emergency.[17] So why not ingest an IV before you get injured or sick.

Hydrating while you are exhibiting early signs of getting sick is important. I have found if I sneeze for no reason, it is an early sign that in 2 days I am going to catch a cold. It is easy to shrug off, but if you can observe what signs you exhibit before you get sick then you can be proactive and not get as sick. So, when I see these signs I will take extra vitamins and a few extra glasses of water.

Coconut water and sport drink marketing will talk about isotonics. Isotonic is a salt water ratio that means there is 23% salt in the liquid.[22] Which coincidently your blood is the same ratio of 23% salt. Your bodies blood will try to maintain at all costs that your blood remains at 23% salt. This is to maintain your blood level to be at a pH of 7.2. If your pH drops it will pull the minerals from your bones to maintain balance. Your body will sacrifice bone strength to maintain blood health.[18]

Low Humidity and Flying

Traveling, especially if you are flying, is a very good time to super hydrate with an IV drink. When flying, it is very distracting and sometimes tense. Add the feature of when you are inside of a plane it will have a low humidity. Low humidity dries out your respiratory track which is one of your defenses to combating the flu.[23] Low humidity is devoid of water in the air, so this environment will leech water from you.[24] The ideal humidity for humans is 40-70%. However, on an airplane humidity levels can be 10-20%.[25] Airplanes have low humidity to minimize the condensation that would accumulate at high altitudes.

When you are dehydrated your body will be weak and not have the resources to flush the bugs out from the recycled air. I have personally found that when I am sick my body will demand 3 times the amount of water than I usually ingest daily. If I do not keep up with that pace the symptoms will get worse and I will be sick for days. When I do keep the pace, I will stay ahead of the symptoms getting worse and I will not get a full-blown illness. So, I add a little more salt to my water, and when you are hydrated like this you do not have to go wait in line in the back of the plane as much.[26]

Chemicals in the Water

When I ask my clients what their source of water is, many will say tap water and that they filter it. Tap water has very little minerals and has chlorine and fluoride. The molecule chlorine and fluoride are chemicals the body has little use for.[19] Fluoride is now quite controversial in that it should be consumed. It has shown to prevent cavities in some cases and at the same time will increase your chance of a hard attack. Fluoride's intention is to harden the teeth but what it also does is harden internal organs. Anyways, what are your teeth made of fluoride or minerals?[27] I am voting minerals, so I make a point to ingest minerals instead of fluoride for my teeth health.[31]

Fluoride and chlorine are a poison that the body will eject quickly. Of course, the amount will take will not harm you today, however, over a period there may be an accumulation effect. Tap water is also missing salt. Salt helps the body absorb water.[28]

The body does allow for trace amount of chlorine and fluoride but when these levels are reached the body will expel them. Therefore, if you drink a bunch of tap water you are also continually going to the bathroom because the body is not absorbing it and it doesn't want it. Try observing drinking a bunch of tap water, now wiggle your stomach around and hear the sloshing sound. This means the water is not absorbing. I will add a pinch of salt to my spring water and there is no sloshing sound at all. This may mean the water is truly absorbed.

So, all water is not created equal. Just because water is clear and flowing does not mean it is health. Distilled water is devoid of minerals. It is often used in experiments and then minerals are added to it. Distilled water seeks an electrical balance, so it is often a mineral stealer.[14]

Reverse osmosis is like distilled water and its purpose is to remove chemicals like fluoride from the water. However, distilled and reverse osmosis are clean from chemicals, but they leave the water molecule in a weakened state. The water molecule will seek balance and pull in minerals from somewhere else. If you are the one drinking it, the imbalanced water molecule will pull the minerals from your bones. This is a variable of osteoporosis. So, it is likely that when the water leaves you it is more electrically balanced then when you first ingest it. A river cleans the water by the rocks donating minerals to the water. This electrically balances the water molecule. So too will your bones give up minerals to balance the water molecule.[15]

In grocery stores you may see a water bottle fill up station. This may be a reverse osmosis machine. The source of the water is tap water and then they use a reverse osmosis machine. The main thing to look for is more minerals and less chemicals.

Alternative Sources for Water

Tests have also show that "activated carbon" filters get rid of some of the chlorine and none of the fluoride.[29]

A low-tech way of turning your tap water into better health water is to filter your water, put it in a pitcher, and let the chemicals evaporate, then add minerals. I don't know how long or how much chemicals evaporate over a period, but, better than nothing. I just consider tap water as a poison and has very little purpose. I don't even like watering my garden with it because I think it strips the organic label from the garden because I am adding chlorine and fluoride chemicals. I have talked to plant nursery's and they say in late-summer when they need to water their plants with tap water 1/3 of them will die.

Well water seems to be good as it is ground water that gets filtered by the ground. However, it may still have some chemicals from pollution and it should be checked to see if it has a good balance of minerals.

The best water to drink is spring/artesian water. Spring water and well water are 2 completely different entities. Spring water flows out of the ground and well water you need a pump to get it out of the ground. Spring water is water that has never touched the surface. According to www.primarywaterinstitute.org they say the difference between well water and spring water is that spring water is missing radioactive isotopes. Most surface water is contaminated with these radioactive isotopes from nuclear testing. When granite is compressed under pressure 40% of it will turn into water. The centrifugal force of the spin of the earth creates this pressure on the granite crust. Wherever there is a thin area in the earth crust the spring water will be pushed through. Primary Institute will drill these areas about 1000-3000 feet down to open these channels and a geyser of water will come out and they will tap it. This is how some rivers and lakes are created. If a lake does not have a mountain stream feeding it is likely a spring fed lake. I have seen ponds above sea level creating streams. Some of these springs are amongst the best source of water. They are minerally rich and not contaminated. In the Puget Sound area, you will see ponds, lakes, and streams all over. If you look at a map you can see that the west part of Puget Sound has been stretched. The crust is thin, and many lakes and ponds are everywhere. We should be tapping these springs and feeding them into our homes. It is estimated that there is 2 times the amount of water under the crust than on the surface. Nearly an unlimited supply of mineral rich clean water is all around us. We need to tap in.[20]

The third source of water I suggest is the $3000 water machines. These machines can clean the water and change the pH. You can make 2.0 - 11.0pH. Many people know about alkaline water which is 7.0 – 14.0 pH and acidic water is 0 – 6.9 pH. Some of the people who use these water machines will drink 8.0 - 9.0 pH water. There is some controversy about this. In either extreme of the pH scale things burn. You got bleach on the acidic side and hydrogen peroxide on the alkaline side, they both burn. Ideally it is recommended to be drinking 7.0-7.4 pH water. It has been found that people with cancer will have a low pH. Perhaps a treatment of 8.0 pH in this case may help. However, one should go slow when you change your pH. I add minerals to my water and when other people do it they have a disgusting reaction to it. Shocking your pH is a little unsettling at first and is an acquired taste. If you think mineral water is disgusting, then you may have a severely low pH. This means you are acidic, and when you are too acidic is it just as the word describes "acid". Acid breaks things down and if you are in a state of being too acidic for a long period of time your body thinks it is dead and will start to assist you in breaking your body down to return you to the earth. Parasites will start to take over and begin to thrive and start eating your body and excreted their wastes which can create strange diseases like dementia?[30]

Fungus and mold will assist in the breakdown which creates more inflammation, which is the foundation of cancer. When we ingest alkaline water rich in oxygen this kills parasites and fungus thus killing

Tap Water

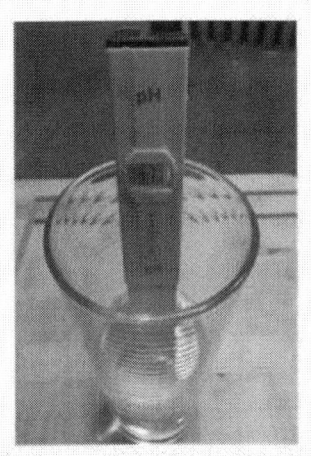

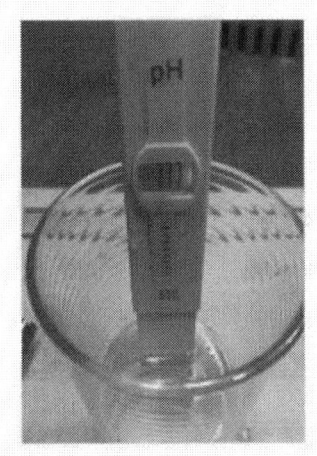

Starting at 6.77pH added 12 drops of Concentrace Minerals Ending at 7.77pH

Spring Water

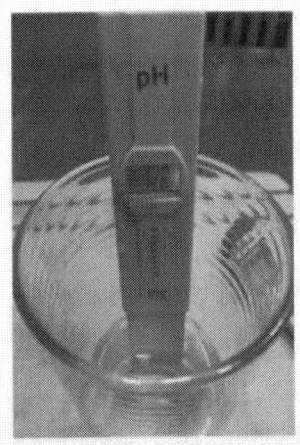

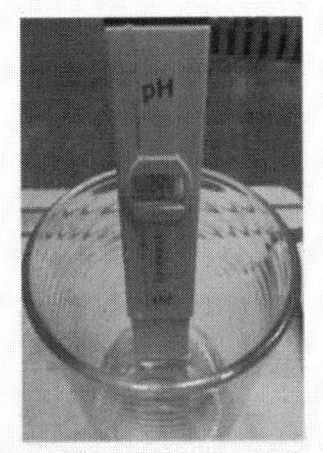

Starting at 7.28pH added 12 drops of Concentrace Minerals Ending at 7.94pH

cancer. So, it may be possible ingesting pure uncontaminated 7.35 pH water may prevent cancer.[21]

I conducted my own experiment with my digital pH reader. I started with tap water and measured it. I was curious what the pH of the sources of water were and how much minerals it took to climb the pH up to 8.0pH.

I then measured spring water. Both has equal amounts of 7 ounces of water. I added 2 drops of ConcenTrace Minerals Product (a concentration of liquid minerals).

pH	Tap Water:	Spring Water:
Start:	6.72	7.28
2 Drops	6.94	7.33
4 Drops	7.04	7.70
6 Drops	7.38	7.75
8 Drops	7.53	7.81
10 Drops	7.70	7.88
12 Drops	7.77	7.94

So, in Seattle, WA the tap water measures below 7.0pH and is already acidic. This tap water was already filtered. The spring water is from a local artesian spring and is not filtered. So, I make the drive to the spring every month.

Dehydration

Stiff joints over a period can be due to dehydration. This can cause inflammation because the muscles do not have the "lubrication" to fluidly bend. When a muscle is dehydrated it will stick to itself and remain stuck in that position until they are hydrated. It is almost better to sit in one place being hydrated rather than moving around all day being dehydrated.

"I must have slept wrong". Actually, you always sleep that way. What you did was you went to sleep dehydrated. You were in a certain position and your muscle stuck to itself. You then turned suddenly and pulled the muscle. So "sleeping wrong" is really you pulled a muscle in your sleep because you were dehydrated.

"Eccentric exercise performed when an individual is dehydrated may exacerbate the skeletal muscle damage because of reduced intracellular water. Eccentric muscle activity with decreased intracellular water during dehydration has been theorized to lead to structural, contractile, and enzymatic protein denaturation.

Dehydration negatively affects muscle performance by impeding thermal regulation, altering water movement across cell membranes, and interfering with actin-myosin cross-bridge formation." [1, 2] - Hargreaves M, Febbraio M

Whether you are a professional athlete or one who is at a computer all day, it is important to hydrate. When we are in excessive heat, coming down with an illness, or in a challenging workout it is important to hydrate because your body is going to assume you are going to hydrate. So, the bodies system is going to move heat out of the body through perspiration. If you are in one of these activities it is important to drink more water than usual. 3

According to, "Biochemical, Physiological and Molecular Aspects of Human Nutrition." Athletes commonly have tight muscles, as do people who are under stress. Tightness from stress usually is experienced in the upper shoulders, neck and around the jaw. Chronically tight muscles lose their flexibility and might become painful to the touch. Mineral deficiency, especially magnesium, can lead to muscle tightness, twitching and maybe even restless leg syndrome at night. A lack of electrolytes, such as sodium, interferes with nerve conductance to muscle fibers and results in tightness and spasms. Poor blood circulation hampers the minerals, electrolytes and water getting to muscles, which can cause symptoms. Other conditions that can cause muscle tightness include pregnancy, diabetes, infections and poorly fitting shoes.[5] -LiveStrong.com

Structured Oxygen Water

In my quest for optimum health I ran into a group that supported Langenburg Technologies. They create oxygen water that is micro-clustered. This micro-clustering is about creating a very small water molecule that the body can easily absorb. This water molecule is packed with oxygen thus able for your body to easily and quickly absorb water and oxygen.

I have drunk a few gallons of this oxygen water. It feels like a super detox. It feels like my body is a piece of coral and water is passing through it very easily. The feeling of sludge and chemicals are being removed and at the end of the day I have a little more energy.

"It began with me looking at the water in Germany, which is full of bacteria and chemicals. I paid more and more attention to it, and then, the water became my passion," says inventor of Langenburg Oxygen Water Max Langenburg.

The basic concern of the human body on a cellular level is to get nutrition in and wastes out. If we become dehydrated or our body becomes an anaerobic (oxygen deficient) environment, several undesirable yet preventable events can take place.

Waste products and toxins can no longer be easily flushed out by the body. Without enough water, metabolic processes and nutrient transport are extensively hindered. Tissue dehydration begins to perpetuate the first signs of premature aging. The immune system stops working properly because communication between the body's 100 trillion cells and 100 billion brain neurons becomes atrophied or suffocated by insufficient oxygen and gradually increasing toxic accumulations.

Our bodies are equipped with an intelligent immune system capable of recognizing and preventing foreign bodies from entering a cell membrane if oxygen is well supplied. Along with helping to maintain a healthy immune system, Langenburg Oxygen Water helps detoxify and eliminate harmful substances and restore good communication between our cells. Healthy levels of oxygen also enable our bodies to burn fat instead of glucose, thus preventing the buildup of lactic acid in the muscles.

The right pH balance is also an integral preparation to many aspects of our health - it allows the body to be in its most prime state to absorb available oxygen, vitamins, minerals and hydration from food and drink. A body with enough oxygen and a healthy pH balance is an unsuitable environment for anaerobic pathogens to flourish.

We begin with water from our natural, protected Oregon water source and sample it for quantitative analysis in preparation for purification and processing.

All harmful toxic elements are removed.

The water is balanced to ensure an optimum pH of approximately 7.7.

We structure the water so that its liquid crystalline and energetic properties are restored.

We then restore optimum oxygen levels (in biochemically superior forms) naturally, and by a process which keeps the oxygen's bio-availability and health benefits stable upon opening the bottle. The oxygen does not escape from the bottle as a gas form of oxygen would almost immediately, and as it does in other oxygenated waters. Our oxygenation process also renders those same benefits intact regardless of temperature or light conditions.

Zeta Potential: *This property is known chiefly as the repulsive force which causes the retained electrostatic charges of minute colloidal particulates to remain in suspension. Our water has a high zeta potential (electrostatic charge), which causes the water molecules to repel rather than bind together. In this way the water maintains its small, microcluster structure allowing the cells to more readily absorb the oxygen contained within.*[6]

[I have become a distributer for the Langenburg products if you would like to order some of the products shoot me an email at steps2light@yahoo.com]

According to the 1931 Nobel Prize winner, Dr. Otto H. Warburg, who devoted his life to the study of the causes of cancer, "all normal cells have an absolute requirement for oxygen, but cancer cells can live without oxygen - a rule without exception. Deprive a cell 35% of its oxygen for 48 hours and it may become cancerous." Dr. Warburg has made it clear that the root cause of cancer is oxygen deficiency, which creates an acidic state in the human body. Dr. Warburg also discovered that cancer cells are anaerobic (they do not breathe oxygen) and cannot survive in the presence of elevated levels of oxygen, as found in an alkaline state.[7]

Cancer cells cannot live in an environment rich in oxygen. At a pH above 7.4 cancer cells become dormant and at a pH of 8.5 cancer will die while healthy cells live. Cancer and some diseases are electron stealing which means your issues will persist while in an oxygen deprived state.[8]

Dr. Jerry Tennant, MD talks about in his book "Healing is Voltage" how water at 7.35 pH kills cancer. The pH of water means potential hydrogen. Hydrogen is energy, so this can also be read as potential energy. Our bodies live off energy in the simplest of form. When we eat and drink it is important our consumables have energy. When our consumables lack minerals, oxygen, and energy our bodies do not know what to do with this material. So allergic type reactions are created like ulcer colitis, leaky gut, rosacea, eczema, breathing problems and the like.[9]

The pH of our water and our bodies is important to maintain voltage for our health. We are electrical being and we need to consume things that are high in voltage. When we are consuming things in the alkaline state we are receiving voltage to repair our bodies. When we stay in an acidic state and consume acidic items we will be losing energy.

When water is at a pH of 7.35 we are consuming -20mV of energy. When we consume water pH at 7.45 this will have -20mV of energy. To create new cells to repair an injury the voltage to create this is -50mV, that is water at 7.88pH. If your body is not consuming enough energy to repair itself then it will be in a constant chronic inflammatory state. Symptoms can be chronic fatigue, and/or your body just does not resolve or repair anything. The more voltage the body has the more oxygen will be absorbed into the water molecule. When we consume electron stealing items this will take energy away from us. Antioxidants help in assisting on neutralizing free radicals which takes energy away from us. Food items will alternate between acidic and alkaline. It is important to do both, however at the end of the day you want the total of alkaline to win out. If acidity wins out your body will be predominantly in an acidic state. If in a constant acidic state your body thinks it is dying so it will start breaking down the body and things like fungus and other pathogens will take over. Some believe that cancer is a fungus, this will help the body breakdown and return to the earth. So, if you would like to keep living, keep your body consuming at least 7.4pH water.[10,11,12]

Walking Barefoot absorbs Energy

The earth is a large electromagnet device and will donate electrons to you. By walking barefoot on the earth, you will absorb electrons. If you are wearing shoes you will be insulated from the earth and you will not absorb electrons.

If you take a quartz crystal and squeeze it with a pair of pliers, it will emit electrons. This is called a piezoelectric effect. Our muscles are piezoelectric crystals. Thus, when we exercise, our muscles create electrons. The muscles are also rechargeable batteries. Thus, the movement of our muscle's re-charge our muscle batteries. Exercise is a major way the body acquires electrons.[13]

"Healing is Voltage" by Dr. Jerry Tennant

Chapter Sixteen

The StretchFlex Technique

A Stretch and Flex a day keeps the Surgeon away

Opposing Muscle Groups
Cause and Effect

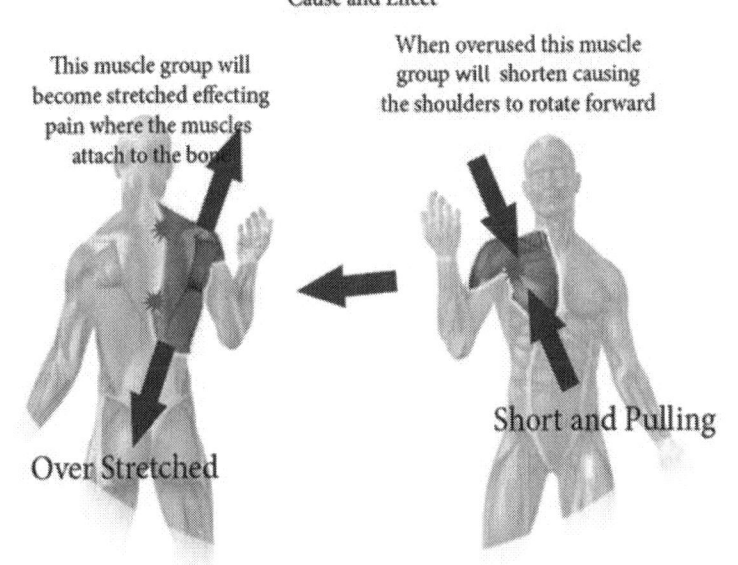

This muscle group will become stretched effecting pain where the muscles attach to the bone

When overused this muscle group will shorten causing the shoulders to rotate forward

Over Stretched

Short and Pulling

The StretchFlex Technique can be overlaid onto any stretch that you already know, and it just requires one more step. When you do a normal stretch notice where the pain is. The pain is the tight muscle being stretched. While you are at the end of the stretch, focus on precisely where the pain is located and then begin to flex that muscle in the opposite direction. Note: One always needs resistance to flex the muscle into something like an elastic band, door frame, bench, or friend holding your arm or leg. Flexing into the air sort-of works but it is best to flex into an item. It is an easy technique to do, to the observer it may look like you are just doing the traditional stretch. If you can do multiple slight little flexes and stretches you will notice significant improvements and have greater range of motion and less pain with any appendage.

Opposing Muscle Groups
Sharing the same appendage

This Muscle Group
Brings the Arm Backwards

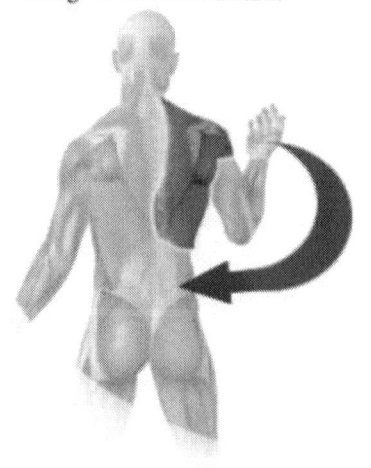

This Muscle Group
Brings the Arm Forward

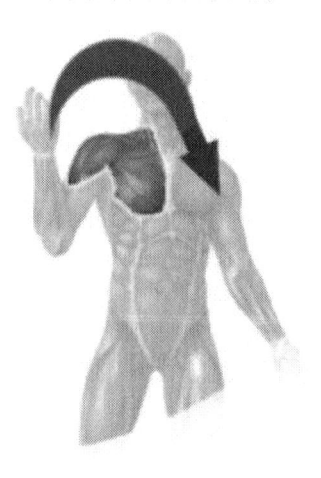

If you are doing the traditional hamstring stretch where you straighten your leg over a bench...stretch the back of your hamstring and then keep your leg straight and flex the painful muscle downward into the bench. The same technique can be applied when stretching the pectoral chest muscle. Against a door frame, stretch your arm backwards and when you feel that it is as far as you can stretch then flex the muscle forward focusing on flexing the painful chest muscle.[1]

If the back of your neck is overstretched, and most peoples are, while lying on a bed tuck your chin and flex your head backwards into the bed. This will shorten and strengthen the back of your neck muscles which will help one have fewer headaches.

The StretchFlex Technique will greatly improve your range of motion and you will have less pain doing it which will likely lead you to doing more stretches.

It is important to flex and stretch every appendage in both directions. Pain is usually from an overstretched muscle. However, just focusing on overstretched muscles is only half the problem. By working both sides of the motion you will increase the integrity of that joint. This is often what carpal tunnel, computer mouse arm, headaches, and arthritis are all about...the joint is being pulled too often in one direction and pain is the indicator that the appendage needs to be balanced.

The whole walking stride is the only time we are stretching and flexing. In Step Point 1 when you lift your foot before your heel hits the ground you are flexing the front of your shin (Tibialis Anterior Muscle), after Step Point 4 you are pushing off your toe and flexing your calf muscle. This action can be the StretchFlex Technique. Also, in the Step Point 1 you are opening your arch and between Step Point 2 and

3 you are then flexing your arch. When you are using Step Point 1 and 2 you are flexing your outside leg muscles and when you are using Step Point 3 and 4 you are using your inside leg muscles.

So, in a single stride you are using the StretchFlex Technique 3 times. Any lack of stretching and flexing in any of these areas will create all the previous ailments that this book is about. Exercising the full range of motion in any appendage will help prevent and maintain all your joints.

A similar massage technique that is just like the StretchFlex Technique is the Muscle Energy Technique. I like calling things by what they do, so in the name, the average person knows what is going on. When you are actively walking you are doing the Muscle Energy Technique and the StretchFlex Technique. It is flexing a muscle group one way while stretching the opposite muscle group. And then they take turns. So that there is a constant trading of back and forth of stretching and flexing. An imbalance happens, or potential injury is created if there is not a 50-50 share of stretching and flexing.[2]

Sometimes muscles can be so tight that they are not stretchable. A massage 2-4 times a month will help loosen that muscle and then the StretchFlex Technique will be easier to do.

Using the StretchFlex Technique may prevent arthritis and any other potential injuries which will hopefully keep you off the operating table.

The StretchFlex Technique only requires about 2-5 minutes a day. After about 1-2 weeks you may notice some significant improvement. I think this technique is 10 times more effective than just stretching and is less painful.

By being aware of how to maintain your body and know when you are about to hurt yourself, which will lead to better health and overall greater spiritual awareness.

Pain is a warning light to let you know something is in trouble. Often people will ignore the pain or use something to suppress it. But if you use pain as a guide to repair yourself you may now have a different relationship with pain. Pain is telling us what to do. When you move a scar tissued injury around there will be some pain. If you slowly flex where the pain is, notice how it goes away. Keep moving your appendage around and find the next painful area. Watch how it goes away once you flex it. Sometimes my left shoulder will get tight and I can get a headache from it. As I slowly flex my arm and shoulder where the pain is. The pain will travel to my elbow. I do the StretchFlex Technique with my elbow and the pain in my neck is gone. So really my shoulder pain was due to my tight elbow. Often where the pain is, is not where the problem is. In my case, my tight arm muscles where pulling on my shoulder muscles. When I loosened up my elbow the shoulder pain tension is gone. This is also the importance of viewing the body from a distance. Often, we look at things through a microscope and only deal directly at the pain center.

So, pain is caused by lack of awareness. When we don't pay attention to ourselves we get in trouble. Pain is helping you to directly take care of an issue. When it comes to rehabilitating an injury, we need more body awareness. When you flex the painful muscle, you are being aware of your body. This alone is the basis for some basic Energy Work 101. Which is paying attention to the body and breathing. Add flexing to the attention and you will have some new skills on fixing your body yourself.

Conclusion

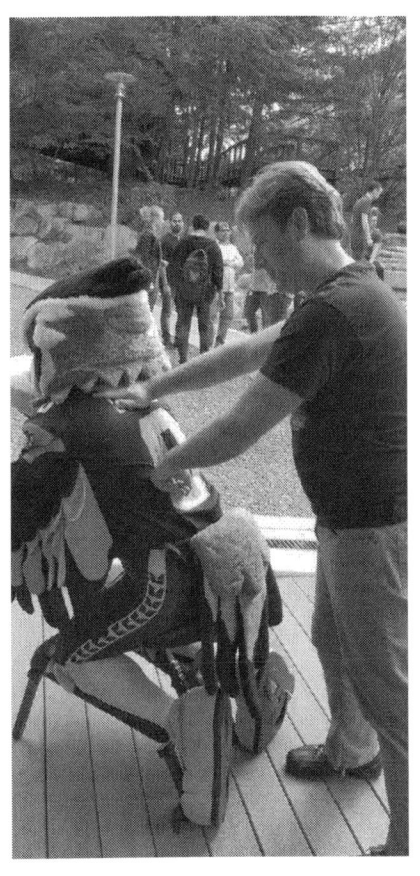

So, as you can see there is a lot going on in every step we take. Taking our time to pay attention to all the tiny aspects of our life can start to explain what is going on in life. Reflecting on how you live your life and slowing it down, we can then start to diagnose what we are doing right and wrong. I believe there are solutions everywhere and that most world, personal, and relationship problems can be solved. Typically, they are so simple that it is unfathomable. I hope this super detail focus of Walking Naturally will help you with your walk and perhaps see that if you slow the world down a little bit you can be responsible for yourself and empower your own healing.

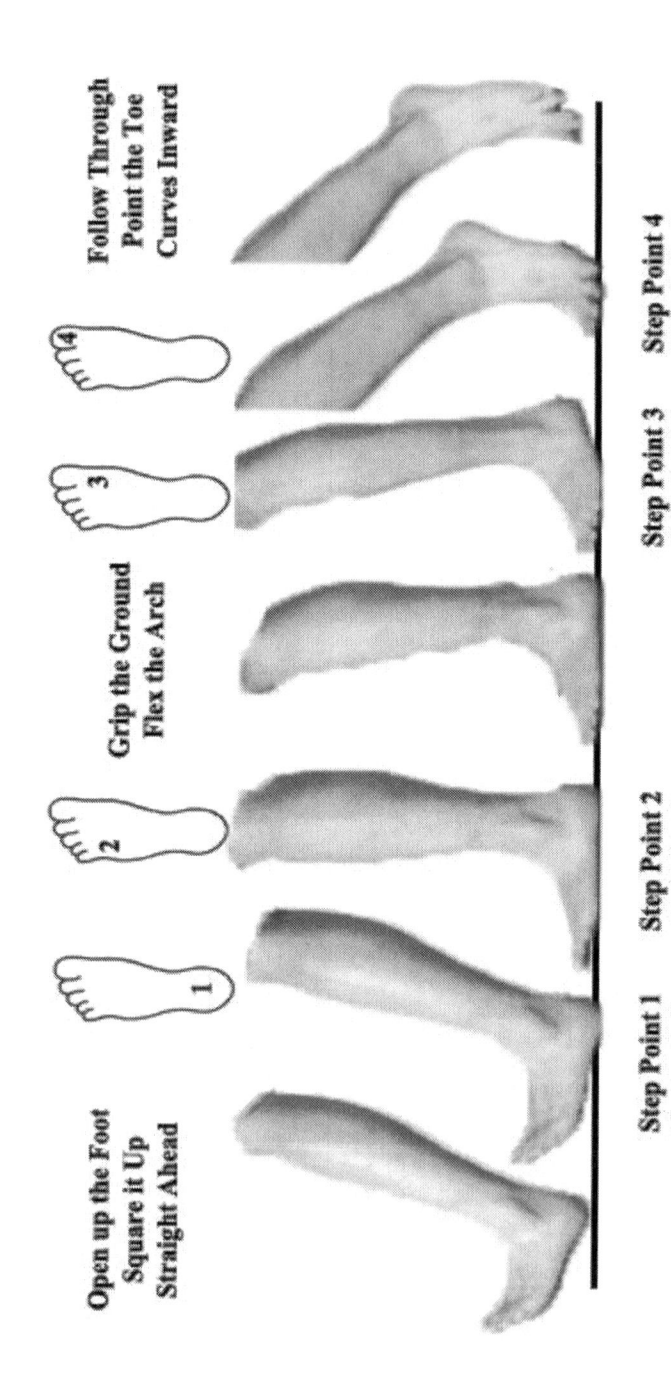

Open up the Foot	Grip the Ground	Follow Through
Square it Up	Flex the Arch	Point the Toe
Straight Ahead		Curves Inward

Step Point 1   Step Point 2   Step Point 3   Step Point 4

The General Group of Muscles Used

Front Leg   Outside Leg   Outside Leg   Transition   Inside Leg   Inside Leg   Rear Leg

The Four Steps Quick Guide from the book *Walk Away Aches & Pains* by Jacob B. Caldwell, LMT

Notes

Chapter One – Range of Motion of the Ankle is Equal to the Range of Motion of your Hip

1. Range of Motion - https://medical-dictionary.thefreedictionary.com/range+of+motion
2. https://medical-dictionary.thefreedictionary.com/yoga
3. https://en.wikipedia.org/wiki/Tibialis_anterior_muscle
4. https://www.merriam-webster.com/dictionary/inflammation
5. https://www.ncbi.nlm.nih.gov/pmc/articles/PMC5668469/
6. https://www.webmd.com/fitness-exercise/guide/achilles-tendon-injury#1
7. *https://draxe.com/sciatic-nerve-pain/
8. https://www.health24.com/Medical/Arthritis/About-Joint-Pain-Arthritis/7-everyday-things-that-could-be-damaging-your-joints-20150109
9. https://www.ncbi.nlm.nih.gov/pubmedhealth/PMHT0024961/
10. https://www.spine-health.com/conditions/lower-back-pain/pulled-back-muscle-and-lower-back-strain
11. https://www.healthline.com/human-body-maps/gastrocnemius-muscle#1

Chapter Two – Toes Forward

1. https://www.pexels.com/photo/metal-ball-reflection-reflections-36710/
2. https://en.wikipedia.org/wiki/Lateral_rotator_group
3. https://en.wikipedia.org/wiki/Medial_compartment_of_thigh
4. https://www.massagemag.com/fixing-strain-patternsbefore-they-become-pain-patterns-1891/

5. https://draxe.com/sciatic-nerve-pain/
6. https://www.spine-health.com/conditions/lower-back-pain/causes-lower-back-pain
7. https://www.ncbi.nlm.nih.gov/pubmed/21665125
8. https://www.sportsinjuryclinic.net/treatments-therapies/foot-biomechanics-gait-analysis/overpronation

Chapter Three – The Four Step Points

1. https://orthoinfo.aaos.org/en/diseases--conditions/shin-splints
2. http://www.footmech.co.uk/common-podiatry-conditions/leg/shin-splints/
3. http://www.footmech.co.uk/common-podiatry-conditions/leg/shin-splints/
4. https://www.acatoday.org/Patients/Health-Wellness-Information/Back-Pain-Facts-and-Statistics
5. https://www.mayoclinic.org/symptom-checker/low-back-pain-adult/related-factors/itt-20009075
6. https://www.ncbi.nlm.nih.gov/pubmed/23246998
7. https://draxe.com/shin-splints/
8. https://draxe.com/plantar-fasciitis/
9. https://www.webmd.com/fitness-exercise/understanding-plantar-fasciitis-basics

Chapter Four – Grip the Ground – No more Falling Arches

1. https://www.healthline.com/human-body-maps/abductor-hallucis-muscle#1
2. https://www.foot.com/foot-conditions/over-pronation/
3. https://www.verywellhealth.com/high-arched-feet-1337684

4. https://www.coasttocoastam.com/photo/category/Coast-to-Coast-AM/?photo_id=66171#66171/Beyond-Belief-Preview-Joel-Wallach
5. https://www.pexels.com/photo/gray-bridge-and-trees-814499/
6. https://ottawafootclinic.com/practice-areas/abductor-hallucis-strain/
7. https://www.drdavidgeier.com/is-running-bad-for-your-knees/
8. https://www.ncbi.nlm.nih.gov/pubmedhealth/PMHT0024679/
9. https://www.mayoclinic.org/diseases-conditions/osteoarthritis/symptoms-causes/syc-20351925

Chapter Five - The 3 Axes

1. https://www.mayoclinic.org/diseases-conditions/spinal-stenosis/symptoms-causes/syc-20352961
2. https://www.health.harvard.edu/staying-healthy/take-a-deep-breath
3. https://www.psychologytoday.com/us/blog/your-neurochemical-self/201106/shallow-breathing
4. https://www.drweil.com/health-wellness/body-mind-spirit/stress-anxiety/breathing-three-exercises/
5. https://www.ncbi.nlm.nih.gov/pmc/articles/PMC2852989/

Chapter Six – Walking Activates Health

1. https://www.doctorshealthpress.com/general-health-articles/foot-reflexology-benefits/
2. https://www.takingcharge.csh.umn.edu/explore-healing-practices/reflexology/what-does-research-say-about-refloxology
3. https://www.organicfacts.net/health-benefits/other/benefits-of-reflexology.html
4. https://www.nidcd.nih.gov/health/balance-disorders

5. https://www.prevention.com/health/a20497906/what-aging-does-to-your-feet/
6. https://www.takingcharge.csh.umn.edu/explore-healing-practices/reflexology/how-does-reflexology-work
7. https://www.takingcharge.csh.umn.edu/reflexology
8. https://www.dailymail.co.uk/health/article-2306227/Reflexology-effective-painkillers-conditions-ache-arthritis.html
9. http://www.pureella.com/wp-content/uploads/2010/04/reflexology-foot-chart-lifeologia.jpg
10. https://i.pinimg.com/736x/4d/86/c4/4d86c4616cfc3305407a95aeb5282197.jpg
11. http://www.reflexologyresearch.net/ReflexologyLegsKneesAnklesResearch.shtml
12. https://www.britannica.com/science/growth-hormone
13. http://nymag.com/health/features/46213/index2.html
14. https://www.healthline.com/health/how-to-perform-lymphatic-drainage-massage#effectiveness

Chapter Seven – Walking effects Posture

1. https://ottawafootclinic.com/custom-made-orthotic/
2. http://medical-dictionary.thefreedictionary.com/cross-fibre+friction+massage
3. https://www.mayoclinic.org/symptom-checker/low-back-pain-adult/related-factors/itt-20009075

Chapter Eight – The Core

1. https://www.aurawellnesscenter.com/2011/05/09/yoga-exercises-for-core-muscles/
2. https://draxe.com/psoas-muscle/

3. https://draxe.com/psoas-muscle/
4. https://www.yoganatomy.com/iliacus-muscle/
5. https://www.whattoexpect.com/pregnancy/pregnancy-health/pregnancy-hormones/hpl.aspx
6. https://www.parents.com/parenting/moms/healthy-mom/new-mom-injuries/

Chapter Nine - Posture

1. https://www.healthline.com/health/lordosis
2. https://www.spinemd.com/symptoms-conditions/kyphosis

Chapter Ten – Not all pain is created equal

1. https://www.arthritis.org/about-arthritis/understanding-arthritis/what-is-arthritis.php
2. https://www.amazon.com/Plastic-Bubble-People-Jacob-Caldwell/dp/197568124X
3. http://www.orthop.washington.edu/?q=faculty-profiles/frederick-a-matsen-iii-md.html
4. http://www.orthop.washington.edu/?q=patient-care/articles/arthritis/joints.html
5. Managing Sports Injuries (Fourth Edition), 2011
6. https://www.ncbi.nlm.nih.gov/pubmed/6493092/
7. *Coast to Coast am 6/11/2018* https://www.youtube.com/watch?v=LvuhxBVuc_4&list=RDtAio_zTHWP8&index=23
8. *https://www.betterbones.com/alkaline-balance/why-an-alkaline-diet-makes-sense/*
9. https://www.calmclinic.com/anxiety/signs/muscle-tension

10. https://www.painscience.com/articles/diagnosing-shortness-of-breath.php
11. http://stretchcoach.com/articles/scar-tissue/
12. https://www.builtlean.com/2013/09/17/muscles-grow/
13. Young sb Kwon, M. a. (2004). How do muscles grow?
14. Petrella JK, Kim JS, Mayhew DL, Cross JM, Bamman MM. Potent myofiber hypertrophy during resistance training in humans is associated with satellite cell-mediated myonuclear addition: a cluster analysis. J Appl Physiol. 2008;104(6):1736-42.
15. Schoenfeld BJ. The mechanisms of muscle hypertrophy and their application to resistance training. J Strength Cond Res. 2010;24(10):2857-72.
16. Kraemer WJ, Ratamess NA. Hormonal responses and adaptations to resistance exercise and training. Sports Med. 2005;35(4):339-61.
17. Tipton KD, W. E. (2001). Exercise, protein metabolism, and muscle growth. Int J Sport Nutr Exer Metab, 109-32,.
18. https://www.youtube.com/watch?v=cK5RGA7PE8s
19. https://medlineplus.gov/ency/article/007021.htm
20. http://www.drjeffs.com/homeostasis_and_physical_healing
21. http://www.thebodysoulconnection.com/EducationCenter/fight.html
22. *https://gallatinvalleychiropractic.com/Arthritis.html*
23. https://medical-dictionary.thefreedictionary.com/microtear
24. https://medical-dictionary.thefreedictionary.com/homeostasis">homeostasis
25. https://sciencing.com/homeostasis-affect-ph-level-4565159.html
26. https://www.verywellhealth.com/what-is-bone-on-bone-2552133

27. https://www.jospt.org/doi/abs/10.2519/jospt.2017.7268?code=jospt-site
28. https://www.best-constipation-remedies.com/chronicdehydrationsymptoms.html

Chapter Eleven – Mental Manifesting

1. https://psychologydictionary.org/manifest-goal/
2. https://www.psychologytoday.com/us/therapy-types/acceptance-and-commitment-therapy
3. https://jamesclear.com/akrasia
4. https://www.psychologytoday.com/us/blog/pieces-mind/201207/radical-acceptance

Chapter Twelve – Shoes- The Good, Bad, and the Funny Looking

1. http://exhibits.hsl.virginia.edu/clothes/lady_bound/
2. https://www.webmd.com/pain-management/ss/slideshow-worst-shoes-for-your-feet

Chapter Thirteen – Sports and Recreation

1. http://journals.sagepub.com/doi/abs/10.1177/03635465030310040501
2. https://orthopedicspecialistsofseattle.com/healthcare/injuries/common-ski-snowboard-injuries/
3. https://www.spine-health.com/blog/poor-posture-causing-your-back-pain

Chapter Fourteen - Therapies, Solutions & Exercises for Superior Walking Health

1. https://www.spine-health.com/treatment/chiropractic/chiropractic-treatments-lower-back-pain
2. https://www.ncbi.nlm.nih.gov/pubmed/21036279
3. https://www.ncbi.nlm.nih.gov/pubmed/16517383
4. https://www.spine-health.com/conditions/sciatica/sciatica-treatment
5. https://www.spine-health.com/wellness/massage-therapy/massage-therapy-lower-back-pain
6. https://www.ncbi.nlm.nih.gov/pubmed/25271201
7. http://www.espn.com/blog/seattle-seahawks/post/_/id/15543/russell-wilson-spends-10-hours-per-week-getting-massages
8. http://www.espn.com/blog/pittsburgh-steelers/post/_/id/24375/hydrations-massages-ivs-yoga-what-nfl-players-spend-upwards-of-300000-on-to-stay-young

Chapter Fifteen – What is Water?

1. Hargreaves M, Febbraio M. Limits to exercise performance in the heat. Int J Sports Med. 1998;19:S115–S116.
2. https://www.ncbi.nlm.nih.gov/pmc/articles/PMC1421497/
3. https://www.healthline.com/nutrition/7-health-benefits-of-water
4. https://www.ncbi.nlm.nih.gov/pubmed/1602938
5. https://www.livestrong.com/article/446204-can-drinking-plenty-of-water-a-day-prevent-tight-muscles/
6. https://www.langenburgwater.com/pages/science-in-harmony-with-nature
7. https://en.wikipedia.org/wiki/Otto_Heinrich_Warburg

8. "Healing is Voltage" by Dr. Jerry Tennant p142
9. www.coasttocoastam.com 6/11/18 Dr Joel Wallach
10. "Healing is Voltage" by Dr. Jerry Tennant p51
11. "Healing is Voltage" by Dr. Jerry Tennant p56
12. *Gaia.com "The Truth about Cancer" with Ty Bollinger*
13. "Healing is Voltage" by Dr. Jerry Tennant p57
14. https://en.wikipedia.org/wiki/Distilled_water
15. https://www.healthline.com/nutrition/purified-vs-distilled-vs-regular-water#section4
16. https://www.healthline.com/health/dry-throat#cold
17. https://driphydration.com/ingredients-in-our-iv-drip-treatments/
18. https://www.healthline.com/health/food-nutrition/benefits-of-coconut-water
19. https://www.healthline.com/nutrition/purified-vs-distilled-vs-regular-water#section2
20. https://www.livescience.com/1312-huge-ocean-discovered-earth.html
21. *Gaia.com "The Truth about Cancer"*
22. http://www.innovateus.net/health/what-isotonic-solution
23. http://www.pnas.org/content/early/2009/02/09/0806852
24. https://articles.mercola.com/sites/articles/archive/2014/01/13/low-humidity-health-effects.aspx
25. https://www.bustle.com/articles/51112-5-strange-ways-airplane-travel-affects-your-body-from-headaches-to-zits
26. https://www.everydayhealth.com/healthy-travel/air-travel-and-dehydration.aspx
27. https://www.sciencelearn.org.nz/resources/1796-bone-and-tooth-minerals
28. https://drnatashaturner.com/4-ways-quickly-hydrate-body/
29. https://fluoridealert.org/content/top_ten/

30. https://www.dementiacarecentral.com/aboutdementia/facts/causes/
31. www.Gaia.com "Quest for the Cure for Cancer"

Chapter Sixteen– StretchFlex Technique

1. https://en.wikipedia.org/wiki/Eccentric_training
2. https://en.wikipedia.org/wiki/Muscle_energy_technique

Index

Abductor Hallucis — 34-35,38, 41

Achilles — 54

Achilles Tendonitis/Tendinosis — 6-8, 28

ACL - 23

Acupuncture — 144

Arch — 39

Arch Support — 40-41

Arm Swing - 49

Arthritis — xiv, 90

Adductor Longus, Brevis, Magnus - 13

Ankle Pain — 79

Biking — 127-128

Bursitis — xiv, 17

Bunion — xiv

Cancer — 163

Carpal Tunnel - 91

Chiropractic — 143-144

Chronic Neck Pain — xiv, 69

Cervical Spine - 69

Core Muscle Group – 73-78

Dehydration – 53, 92-93, 102, 151, 159

Distilled Water - 151

Dr. Joel Wallach – 95

Dr. Jerry Tennant – 95, 163, 165

Dr. Otto Warburg – 163

Dr. Max Langenburg – 160-162

Dr. Neil F Neimmak – 100

Dr. Susan Brown – 96

Extensor Hallucis – 30-31

Falling Arches – 21-22, 37, 46

Fluoride - 153

Football – 134-139

Gall Bladder – 57

Gemellus Inferior - 12

Gemellus Superior – 12

Gluteus Maximus – 12

Gluteus Medius – 12

Gluteus Minimus – 12

Gracillis – 12-13

Grounding to the Earth -   141

Headaches – 47, 63

High Arches - 38

Homeostasis – 100

Iliacus – 20

Immune System - 51

Insanity - xiii

Knee Pain – 22

Kyphosis - 86

Lordosis - 85

Low Back Pain – xiv, 33, 78, 113, 136

Lungs - 58

Lymphatic System – 51-53

Massage Therapy – 145-146

MCL - 23

Medical Intuitive – 117

Mid Back Pain – 54

Muscle Energy Technique - 170

Muscle Fatigue – 2

Muscle Pull – 109-110

Nutrition – 95

Orthotics – xvi

Osteoporosis - 47

Osteoarthritis – 89

Overpronation – 21, 30, 87

Oxygen Water - 160

Pain Scale – 103-108

Parasites - 156

Plantar Fasciitis – xiv, 34, 137

Plastic Suit Bubble People - 90

Piriformis – 12

Pituitary Gland – 62, 65

Pregnancy – 78

Psoas – 20

Piriformis Syndrome - 15

Quadratus Femoris - 12

Range of Motion – 1, 4, 54, 56, 97

Reflexology – 56-64

Reverse Osmosis - 154

Sacral Iliac Joint – 14

Scar Tissue – 69, 92, 198, 101

Scoliosis – xiv, 69

Sciatica – 11, 15-21, 33, 78, 144

Sciatic Nerve – 15, 30, 54-56, 67

Shin Splints – xiv, 30-32

Skating – 32, 130-131

Skiing – 131-133

Spleen – 57

Step Points – 15

StretchFlex Technique – 42, 101, 167-171

Structured Oxygen Water – 208-212

Stomach - 60

Snowboarding – 129-130

Synovial Fluid – 93-94

Tibialis Anterior – 1, 4-6

Yoga – 58, 74, 79, 147-148

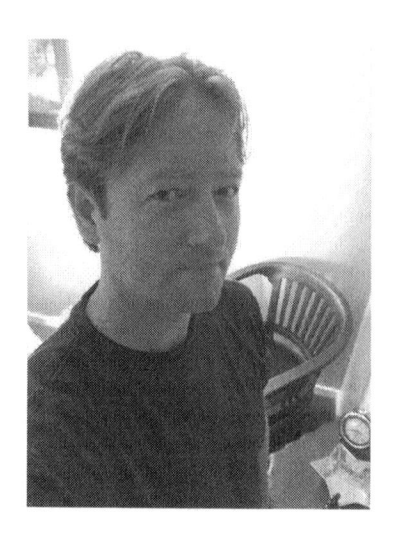

Jacob Caldwell is a Massage Therapist in Seattle. He is passionate about how to help people address the issues they have and will help those that want to heal themselves. In this complex world simplicity is being lost. Jacob has found most of the solutions in the world are quite easy. He is on a mission to help assist in making the world simple.

Walking Correctly can't be any easier, which is the hard part.

www.SeattleMassageBlogger.com

www.SeattleMasssage.co

<u>www.EnergyHealingTherapy.net</u>

Instagram "how2walkcorrectly"

Facebook Fanpage "Seattle Massage Therapy"

Vimeo Videos https://vimeo.com/user2573949

Other Books Authored & Illustrated by Jacob Caldwell

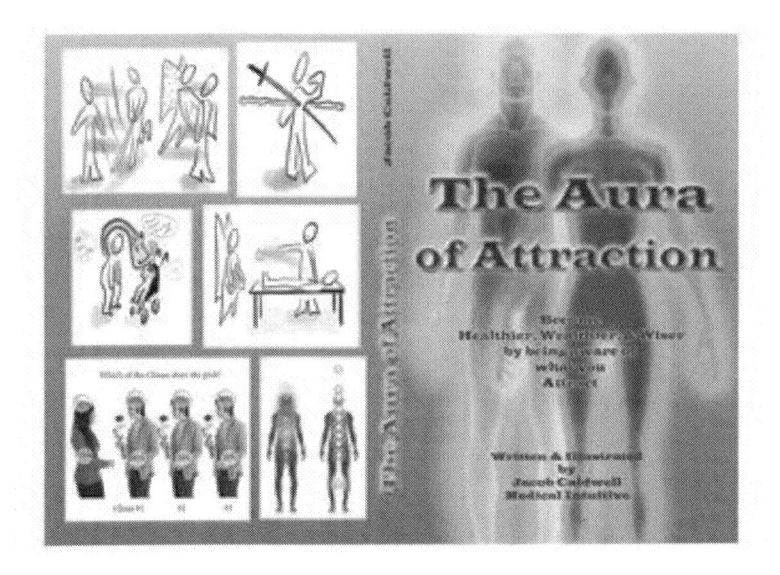

Take the Aura of Attraction Survey
to see what you Attract
Facebook Fanpage "The Aura of Attraction"

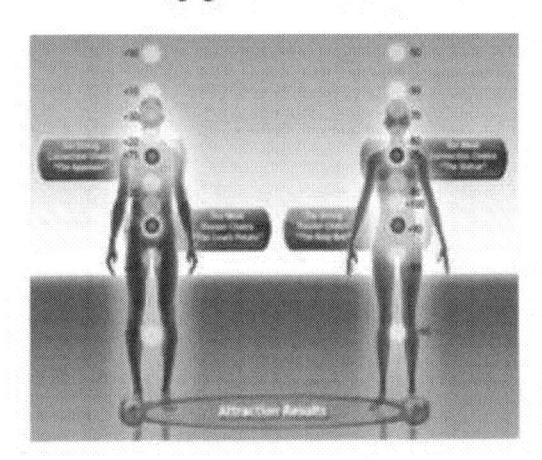

The Aura of Attraction

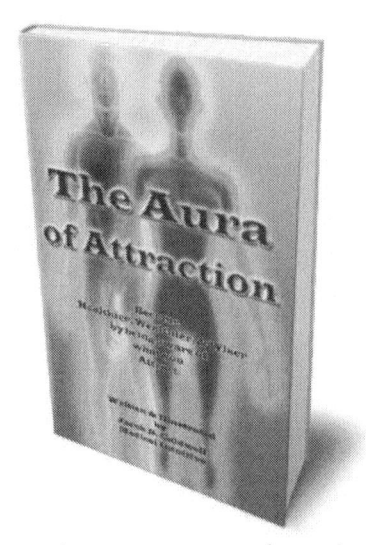

The Aura of Attraction is the collection of illustrated observations from the viewpoint of Medical Intuitive, Jacob Caldwell. He is the author and illustrator of this book. A Medical Intuitive can read people's energy and this book is an illustration on what he has been able to observe. He has been able to turn the invisible visible and demonstrate that the clues of life's guidance are within us. Jacob will help you interpret the daily signs that you receive ad help to find the answers to questions you keep asking. He has been able to see how people create their own disease, circumstances, and good or bad relationships. He has created a book that will help those that want to take the reins of their life and change it for the better. If you are tired of riding the same daily merry-go-round of insanity and you want to get off, then pick up this book and get ready to step out into your true empowerment. Set your life on your terms and fill it with new meaning by being able to interpret the clues that are all around you, to create a happy life.

Billy Has a Learning Disability

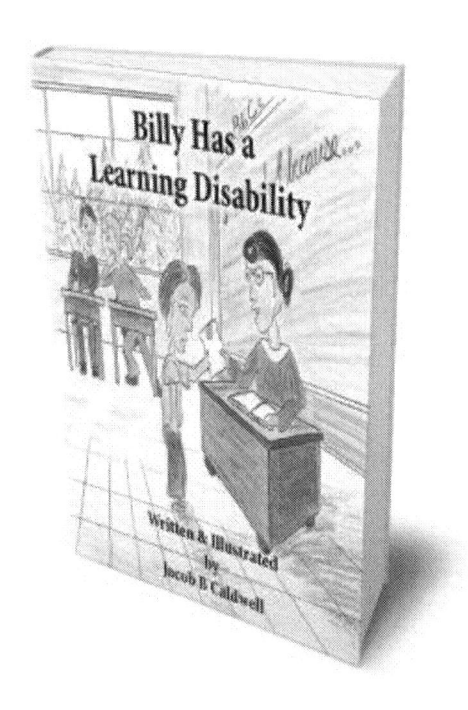

Billy is a boy who has just been told he has a Learning Disability. Billy and his mother work with a tutor who helps him discover that he doesn't have a disability, just that he things differently and has no disability at all. The tutor and Billy work on special tasks that help Billy realize his own Learning Skills.

Plastic Suit Bubble People

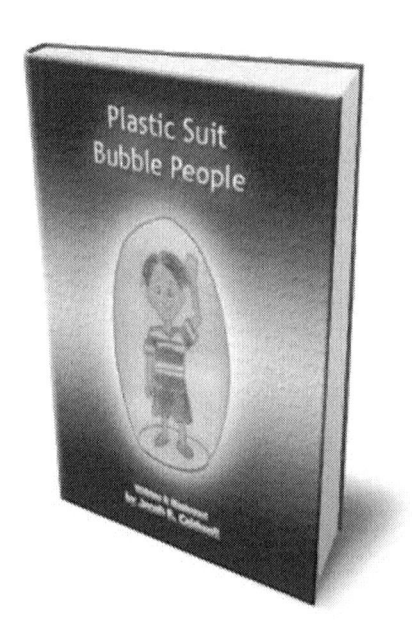

Jacob was inspired to write this book by observing how people walked around and interacted with each other. Sometimes it seems they wished they would rather disappear. Well, what if they could?

In this story an Inventor is able to come up with a Plastic Suit Bubble that can shield people from all the things they fear or don't want to deal with. In the end, perhaps the bubble is more trouble than people can fubble.

Written at the time of the dawning of the internet in 1998. Present day, has our cell phone behavior become the precursor to the Bubble Suit?

"Walk Away Aches & Pains"

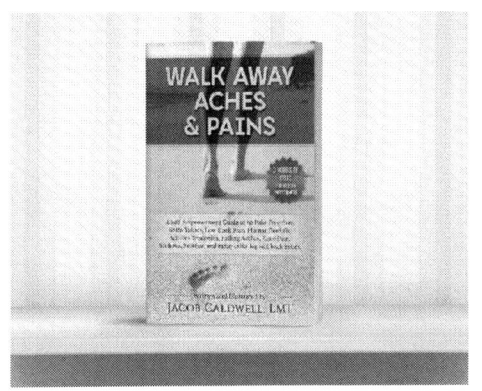

This guide on How to "Walk Away Aches & Pains" is for people who want to be responsible for their own healing. This step by step process of this walking technique will help you alleviate your own leg issues. This is one of the ways to never have to be in a wheel chair or the need to wear orthotics. Learning to walk more naturally will help your overall posture and many of your leg, back, and neck chronic issues may be able to lessen or disappear.

Jacob Caldwell is a Massage Therapist in Seattle who will assist you in empowering you to heal yourself. He has been in practice since 2002 and has been assisting people see that you can alleviate your own symptoms by just walking with more attention.

Continuing Education for Health Practitioners

Copy the Link Below to Start the Receiving Forms

https://forms.aweber.com/form/93/1193346093.htm

Instructor: Jacob Caldwell, LMT

MA000016444

Steps2Light@yahoo.com

Seattle, WA 98199

"Walk Away Aches & Pains" Book	0.5 Hours of CEU
"Walk Away Aches & Pains" Video Series	1.5 Hours of CEU
Apply Knowledge to your Clients	1 Hour of CEU

Total of 3 Hours of CEU's

Links and Sites change my email never will, let me know if you need smething steps2light@yahoo.com

Need A Little More?

Watch the "Walk Away Aches & Pains" Video Series.

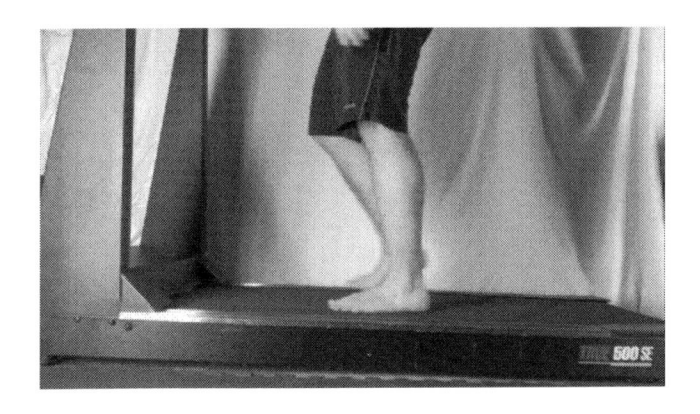

90 Minutes of Video showing how to walk correctly and incorrectly.

It is better to see some of these concepts in motion to fully understand what is going on.

Vimeo.com/ondemand/walkawayachespains

Included in Video Package – Send me a Video of your Walk and I will record a voice over to assist you in making your walk better.

The Full Lesson on how to resolve Shin Splints.

Vimeo.com/ondemand/shinsplintrelief

Bonus Videos

5 Minute Workout for those that Sit or Stand at a Desk

https://youtu.be/Dfjy7e95YQA

How to Sit Correctly

https://youtu.be/Y06-HJq0RO0

StretchFlex Technique

https://youtu.be/-krIweipI-U

Introduction to Pain Free Walking

https://youtu.be/LyVPAqI_E10

Welcome to the Pain Free Walking Video Series

https://youtu.be/nLxUX-v50HE

Made in the USA
Middletown, DE
29 May 2020